Emotional Eating:

Develop Intelligence and Emotional Agility as an Intuitive Advantage and Become Aware of Eating Disorders Learning How to Eliminate Them to Easily Build a Perfect Female Body

rendering of legal, financial, medical or professional advice. The content within this book has been derived from various sources. Please consult a licensed professional before attempting any techniques outlined in this book.

By reading this document, the reader agrees that under no circumstances is the author responsible for any losses, direct or indirect, that are incurred as a result of the use of the information contained within this document, including, but not limited to, errors, omissions, or inaccuracies.

Table of Contents

Introduction

Are you eating more than you should, but feel powerless to stop it? For many people, obesity is a life-long struggle. Despite your best efforts and knowledge, you feel like a constant slave to your appetite. You may not be aware of how often and how much you're eating. You may have an intention to improve, but the sudden waves of excruciating hunger always come back, ruining both your efforts and self-esteem.

If you're experiencing episodes of sudden, unbearable hunger, the reason for that might be more than an empty stomach. If you've picked up this book, you're either aware that you are an emotional eater, or you suspect you are one. Either way, this book studies the complexities of emotional eating, giving you a view of the problem from all sides- physical, emotional, and behavioral.

In this book, you will learn more about what it means to be an emotional eater. You will learn the main causes of emotional eating, and different types of emotional eating. Further, this book explores the deeper emotional issues that lie behind emotional eating.

By reading this book, you will learn how to make a connection between your past experiences, and your present struggles. You will learn how the way you were raised affected your appetite and eating habits.

More importantly, with this book, you will learn how to come to terms with past trauma, and heal in order to become happier, more satisfied, more active, and overall healthier. In this book, we will delve into the reasons why you are using food to cope with feelings, and what you can do to recover from that. Further, we will show you how to become a conscious, mindful eater, who uses food and exercise to obtain health and happiness the right way.

Chapter 1:   What Is Emotional Eating?

Do you feel a sudden urge to eat when there's no sense of physical hunger present? Do you feel compelled to suddenly have a large meal, only to feel overly full, nauseous, and ashamed afterward? If so, the reason for that might be that you are an emotional eater. If you've picked up this book, you are probably aware that you are eating more than you need to, and that your food choices may not be the best.

The Definition of Emotional Eating

Emotional eating is a habit of eating to cope with feelings (Evers et al., 2010). While your intention may be to lift your mood with a satisfying meal, the feeling of guilt is more likely to result from an episode of overeating. Instead of lifting you up, the binge-eating will only make you feel worse.

You, as an emotional eater, are using this habit to ground yourself, calm down, and avoid confronting difficult emotions. But, there's more complexity to emotional eating than just understanding that you are eating to cope. This chapter will explain what is happening inside your mind and body when you face a sudden, irresistible appetite.

Emotional eating closely relates to obesity. There are multiple reasons for this, such as:

- Eating irregular meals;

- Eating large amounts of food once or twice per day;

- Suppressing appetite instead of having regular, healthy meals; and

- Overeating on unhealthy foods;

What Causes Emotional Eating?

Research has shown that there's a significant connection between gaining weight and emotional eating. Still, not much has been done to study emotional eating outside the context of eating disorders. If you haven't been diagnosed with an eating disorder, there might be a couple of different reasons behind emotional eating, such as:

Stress

For women, stress is the main trigger of emotional eating. Initially, stress is the reason to avoid timely, healthy meals, only to overeat at the end of the day. The guilty feeling is frequently present after eating, followed by a sense of shame and negative self-talk.

This happens because eating irregularly causes your body to starve. When your body starves, it will crave carbs and sugary foods as the easiest and fastest source of energy. One of the ways in which you can cope with your feelings instead of turning to food to find comfort is to study stress management.

Boredom

In addition to eating out of stress, people also tend to overeat due to boredom. In this case, you are using the food to distract yourself from the feeling of emptiness and not having anything else to do.

Both men and women tend to choose unhealthy foods to cope with boredom.

Suppressing Feelings

Emotional eating has been mainly viewed as eating as a response to emotional signals. As such, it is mainly a way for you to cope with unpleasant feelings that you unconsciously don't know how to process. The lack of knowledge and skill to process one's own emotions seems to be the main cause of unconscious stress and anxiety that lead to emotional eating. There could be numerous feelings behind emotional eating that you choose to suppress with eating. These feelings include fear, anger, sadness, hopelessness, guilt, shame, and many more. Keeping in mind that inner sensations can cause people to reduce or stop eating, as opposed to over-eating, you can assume that, in your case, the food itself becomes a tool to obtain what you've been missing. It could be a sense of stability, safety, inner peace, love, or companionship. This is the reason why it is important for you to discover the reasons behind your emotional eating.

Stressful Environment

A stressful job, college program, or a stressful relationship can contribute to emotional eating. Being exposed to continuous stress and lacking the time to rest and devote to mindfulness, can cause you to turn to food instead of delving deeper into your own issues. If you think about it, constant deadlines, a stressful job or college program may, indeed, leave insufficient time for you to process your own feelings and reflect on your life the way you should.

Lack of Healthy Food Choices

Living a lifestyle in which you can't find enough time to take care of your own health, often entails insufficient time for healthy eating. A healthy diet requires time to shop and cook your own meals, and if you don't have that time, you might have to resort to widely available fast-food options. The more you consume processed sugars and carbs, the more you'll become addicted to them. This will intensify the cravings when you're in distress. In a triggering situation, the lack of healthy options leaves you with no choice but to reach out for junk food. You might feel like a bowl of salad would lighten your mood, but if the only available option is a bowl of ice cream, you're bound to go for it.

Lack of Physical Activity

A perceived lack of time for physical activity, such as exercise, has a role in emotional eating. Physical activity, aside from benefiting your body, is also crucial for a healthy mind. Being active causes your brain to release endorphins, the happiness hormones. Being physically active also reduces anxiety and the feeling of being overwhelmed. Without sufficient physical activity, you will feel dissatisfied because you aren't spending enough time outside. The feeling of hunger may result from that.

Identity Crisis

Every person goes through challenges and periods of transformation. Using food as a way of coping with an identity crisis can happen to people who are going through big personality changes, but haven't built the skills to cope with them.

Whether you've just finished college, got or lost a job, started a family, or got a divorce, the intense life changes can leave you questioning yourself and your identity. In addition, people naturally evolve and change as they age. Food can sometimes be used to relieve the feelings of uncertainty or to find happiness when the things that used to make you happy no longer do. As you go through natural stages of personal growth, your habits and interests change. If you aren't used to self-reflecting, you won't notice this shift, and you won't open up to explore new interests. The feeling of unfulfillment can cause fear and anxiety, resulting in an increased appetite.

Suppressing Appetite

Many people tend to suppress their appetite during times of stress, only to overeat when the stressful times of the day pass. If you're studying for an exam, you may avoid eating for an entire day, only to spend an entire day binge-eating after the exam. You can read a lot about your emotional eating by just tracking and noting your eating behaviors. For emotional eaters, it is common to, in times of stress, reduce the intake of healthy foods and replace them with candy or fast food. If you're noticing that stress is changing the way you eat, you can work around it. For example, if you know in advance that certain times of your day will be more stressful than others, you can prepare a healthy alternative for your go-to snack.

Social Gatherings

Many find it hard to resist eating while spending time with friends and family. Even if there's a need to diet, people tend to fall under the pressure to participate in group-eating. If the food is a significant part of your friend group's activities and family gatherings, resisting the pressure might be hard.

In this chapter, you've learned a bit more about the definition and the main causes of emotional eating. Regardless of how difficult may seem to break the negative eating patterns, you're anything but hopeless. The following chapters of this book will help you recognize the true causes of your eating problems, and find healthy, self-nurturing ways to cope.

Chapter 2: What Kind of an Emotional Eater Are You?

Knowing what type of an emotional eater you are will help you identify the triggers, and pin-point the areas where you want to improve. This chapter will break down the driving influences behind emotional eating and discover how are you using food to satisfy emotional needs (Konttinen et. al., 2010).

Eating To Celebrate

Do you eat to reward yourself for hard-working efforts? This can happen if you are overworking yourself, and if you are constantly on the go. In this case, you want to treat yourself to something nice, regardless of whether or not it is healthy for you. You may also be using food to find inner peace and boost your self-esteem. If you are a people-pleaser, and you find it hard to say 'no,' you will want to reduce some of the stress that this behavior has caused by eating.

By eating, you are suppressing the thoughts and feelings that you don't want to address. These feelings could be about the fact that there are certain people that you don't like, or that you want or need to set certain boundaries.

To recover from eating as a reward, you need to find better ways to treat yourself. Devote more to acknowledging your qualities, achievements, and efforts. Vocalize and verbalize your achievements, and praise yourself often. Food isn't the only way for you to feel good, and to experience happiness. You can also choose to talk to a friend or a family member, and share the great things that have happened to you.

If you are used to suppressing the feeling of happiness for numerous reasons, you may unconsciously feel like being happy may result in something bad afterward. This can happen often when if you've had a difficult childhood, and you felt like whenever you started to feel happy and joyful, something bad would suddenly happen. If you learned that feeling happy and satisfied is in any way inappropriate or unsafe, you will want to swallow down your happiness. You'll never allow yourself to fully experience it. By learning to acknowledge and experience happiness in mindful ways, you will also reduce the need to eat when you feel happy or when you want to reward yourself.

Eating Away Fear

You could also be eating to cope with the feeling of fear. Fear and anxiety can have a major influence on your appetite. While some people experience a decrease in appetite when afraid, others might feel an increase. Fear also affects your digestion, and can cause an upset stomach, heartburn, indigestion, diarrhea as well as constipation. Fear can drive you to turn to comfort foods that are rich in sugar and carbohydrates, like sweets and fast food.

If you are refusing to face and cope with fears, then they are constantly burning out your mind and body. As a result, you find yourself having to frequently eat in order to recover your energy. In addition to this, you may also be eating to comfort yourself when you're feeling afraid.

Fear and worry are sensations tailored around the need for survival. When you are feeling subconsciously scared and worried, you are questioning whether or not you will be able to cope with the situation. A mundane situation, like being unable to meet your deadline, may trigger the thoughts about losing your job, and compromising your entire life. This exaggerated response of your body, while difficult to cope with, is learned. You can unlearn this response the same way you learned it. So, how to stop eating out of fear?

There are numerous ways in which you can cope with your fear in a healthy way, instead of binge eating. The first thing you want to do, if you think that you might be eating out of fear, is to choose to acknowledge, accept and process your fears. Ignoring them will only make the matter worse.

Next, you want to start tracing the thoughts and feelings that are causing your appetite. If those reasons appear to be related to fear, you want to sit down and note all thoughts and feelings that are currently going through your mind. You want to examine how previous situations are reflecting inside your mind to make you feel constantly afraid.

The next step is to rationalize these fears. Ask yourself these questions.

- Is it really rational for me to fear this?

- What are the chances of this coming true?

You may fear that certain bad things will happen to you without any real factual risk, or feel like you're out of control and have no way of coping with the circumstances. If you unconsciously feel like circumstances might overwhelm you, it may cause resistance to acknowledging the unconscious fears.

If you think that fear is behind your emotional eating, you can go ahead and think about the circumstances that might have contributed to these fears, as well as possible ways for you to cope. However, beneath all this lie deeper self-esteem issues, and issues with feeling insufficiently safe, loved, and comforted. If you don't trust yourself enough, and you don't trust in your abilities to cope with the circumstances that you are facing, you will be constantly in fear. Since you can predict how the events will unravel if they actually happen, you need to trust yourself that you will be capable of coping regardless of what happens.

Last, but not least, you can choose to cope with a feeling without eating. Notice if comforting yourself helps reduce your appetite. Aside from rationalizing and understanding the childhood roots of your fears, knowing how to comfort yourself is also important. The reason that fear caused so much appetite in the first place, is that you were either unwilling, or you didn't have the skill to comfort yourself. So how will you comfort yourself?

Will you turn to a friend for a talk, or you'll have a compassionate conversation with yourself, where you'll state that you believe in your abilities to be fine and to overcome any obstacles? Whichever way you choose, it is a better option than choosing to ignore your fears.

You could have an emotional blockage to processing fears. If you have learned that being afraid is a sign of weakness, you'll want to ignore being afraid, and as a result of that, you are never truly coming to terms with your fears. Your fears are constantly working in the back of your mind, and exhausting your mental and physical energy as a result. You're frequently craving sugars and carbs, and gaining weight as a result of this.

There are numerous fears behind emotional eating, such as fear of loneliness, fear of abandonment, or fear of being inadequate. Behind all of these, there's a lack of unconditional self-love, self-acceptance, and self-esteem.

To detect which of the fears lies behind your binge eating, start by describing the last time you remember feeling calm. Then, describe the last time when you felt a sudden craving to eat.

- What has changed?

- Who did you talk to?

- What did you think about?

- How did you feel?

Eating Away Sadness

Eating to cope with depression and sadness is one of the most frequent reasons for emotional overeating. Learning how to cope with pain and sadness originates in early childhood. It has a lot to do with whether or not, or how were you comforted when you cried, and whether you had an insecure attachment to your caregivers. You might have learned that being sad is a sign of weakness, or that you don't have anyone to rely on when you are sad. If you were taught that you need to be strong and tough in order to survive, you could have missed the opportunity to learn healthy ways to deal with pain. In addition, if you weren't properly comforted when you were sad, you may have formed the belief that there's no use in trying to reach out to anyone, and that you are better off keeping the sadness to yourself.

How to Cope With Sadness

Learning how to cope with sadness will not only help you overcome emotional eating. It will also help you become happier in the long run.

Accept the Sadness

Unfortunate events and pain are a normal part of everyone's life. Building the skills to cope with the pain will make you happier and more productive. To overcome emotional eating, you need to strengthen the ability to cope with the pain. However, you first need to be willing to acknowledge your pain, instead of suppressing it. Be open to acknowledging and honoring your pain.

Learn To Honor Your Pain

Pay attention to your inner self-talk when you are experiencing sadness. Are you prone to blaming yourself for the painful experiences? To begin learning how to cope with pain, start by thinking about the painful situation, and the way it makes you feel. Next, take some time to comfort yourself and explain to yourself that there is no fault, guilt, or shame in feeling pain.

To honor the pain and sadness, take the time to truly become aware of the thoughts that are going through your mind. Don't try to fix the way you feel before you are ready to do it. Instead, take enough time to comfort yourself with positive self-talk and compassion. Express understanding towards your feelings, and acknowledge to yourself that it's okay to feel this way. You have no reason to run from it. Feeling hurt doesn't make you weak. You also don't have to be all right all the time. It is all right to feel sad, and it doesn't say anything about your personality.

Open yourself up to talking about your pain with friends, family, or a therapist. If you haven't learned how to cope with pain in a healthy way, you might feel like the sadness will overwhelm you. It could be one of the reasons why you chose to suppress the pain. You need to be willing to cry and to be honest with yourself without judgment. There are other creative ways to honor your pain that will make you feel comforted and loved. You can think about all the things you would say and do to comfort a friend who was feeling sad, and choose to do the exact same things for yourself. Think about the following strategies:

- What are the nice things you can do to comfort yourself when you are sad?

- Can you take yourself out for a walk?

- Can you rest at home?

- Can you have a nice calming bath or shower?

All of the things that you feel like you would want to do for another person who is hurting, are the exact things that will feel good for you. Being open to acknowledging that you feel hurt, and not judging yourself over it is the first step towards becoming more emotionally intelligent about pain. The next step is to learn to go through life without having to suppress pain. There could be numerous reasons behind your pain, some of them being very serious and dramatic. You may have suffered loss, and you may think that you are unable to live past that loss. You may have suffered trauma. Or, you may be carrying unresolved sadness from earlier life.

Learn To Live While Healing

Whatever the source of your pain might be, the right way to go is to choose to honor your pain while going through life. That means not trying to stop the sadness, or waiting to become happy in order to move on with your life. You can live a healthy life, and spend time with friends and family while you're healing. Acknowledge that you don't have to feel good in order to do a good job. Acknowledge that you don't have to feel good, in order to devote your time to other people and engage in conversations. Acknowledge that you don't have to feel good to go outside, and walk or exercise. An important part of learning how to live with pain is understanding that the pain doesn't have to go away for you continue living a productive life.

The more you acknowledge and deal with your personal pains, the more your struggles with appetite will reduce.

Don't Wait To Improve the Diet

Another important truth to acknowledge is that you don't have to solve all of your emotional problems in order to stop the negative eating patterns. If you enjoy comforting yourself with food, you can always go for leaner, healthier options. Because the purpose of eating in this situation is for you to feel grounded, safe, and comfortable, you can do that with a large variety of foods that are healthy. Soups and broths are healthy, and they are a common choice for comfort food. Instead of ordering takeout, you can have a bowl of nice soup. In addition, if you feel like these comforting rituals are truly beneficial to recovering, you can give more meaning to the food rather than just pouring it down your throat to swallow your feelings. For example, if coping with sadness by staying in and having something nice to eat feels right for you, you can choose to do it, as long as the food choices are healthy and moderate. You can also include other elements that comfort you, such as listening to calming music, watching a funny movie, or reading.

Write The Sadness Down

Journaling is also a great way to deal with sadness. A journal allows you to go in different directions with your thoughts. You don't have to structure them. And you don't have to navigate the journaling process. You can just lay out everything that is bothering you. Simply doing this will relieve a lot of your pressure.

Eating Away Anger

Eating to cope with anger happens because you are trying to ground yourself when you're feeling frustrated and powerless. To overcome this, you can use the situations that make you angry in order to learn something new and improve. Otherwise, you may get lost in the frustration and feelings of shame and guilt. Here's how you can stop eating to suppress anger:

- When you feel frustrated, instead of reaching out for food, you may think about the reasons why the situation went the way it went, and what can you do to help? Prevent it in the future.

- The number one thing that you should do if you suspect that you are eating to suppress anger is to immediately stop the negative behavior. When you catch yourself reaching for the food out of anger, stop it.

- Anger and frustration activate the brain chemicals that put you in a reactive mode. In this situation, you start acting mindless, in some way. For this reason, you need to take a step back, and allow yourself to calm down. This will allow your mind, in particular, the prefrontal cortex which helps you choose the next best step, to do its work instead of acting on impulse. When doing this, make sure that you act with compassion to yourself.

- Next, make sure you look into what you are truly wanting and hoping to achieve. It may be that you are eating when you are angry to experience some self-compassion. There is always a connection between anger and sadness:

  - When you are angry, you are unable to stop yourself from the negative self-talk, and that causes you sadness.

  - When you are angry, to a certain degree, you feel hurt.

  - When you are angry, you are also feeling endangered, powerless, and sad to a certain degree.

When you find yourself in a situation that makes you feel aggravated, and you feel like getting a pint of ice cream, think about who you are truly angry at? Are you angry at the situation, or you are angry at yourself for not knowing the right ways of how to deal with it?

Are you angry about handling the situation in the wrong way, or you are angry at yourself because you were unable to react better? A lot of the time, self-criticism is behind anger. If you think about it, on most days, when you are feeling calm and in a good mood, you are a lot more tolerant and less prone to feeling aggravated. But, when you question yourself and feel insecure about your abilities, you are more likely to get angry.

Before responding to a situation that makes you angry, ask yourself whether you are truly angry with yourself? In the future, is there anything that you want to say or do differently? Answering these questions will help you improve your responses to stressful situations, establish more balanced reactions to anger, and become open to hearing the negative self-talk, so that you can overcome it.

Eating Away Stress

If you are a stress-eater, you will eat when you feel nervous, anxious, tense, worried, panicked, or agitated. You don't want to address the underlying issues, so you turn to food to comfort yourself and suppress overbearing feelings.

How Toxic Self-Criticism Increases Stress and Emotional Eating

A frequent reason behind the stress eating might be to cope with the feeling of guilt and depression. People who cope with anxiety and depression are often inflicted by strong, exaggerated, and irrational self-criticism. When your inner critic starts criticizing you over everything you do, and you feel like you are not good enough regardless of what you do, you may also want to eat as a way to reduce this feeling.

The Role of Constant Pressure And Chronic Exhaustion

Being chronically stressed could also affect your sleep quality. People who are exposed to chronic stress often don't sleep enough, and they are overtired. Being sleep-deprived affects your appetite. As you are depleted both emotionally and energetically, you will crave a lot of sugars and carbs as a way to temporarily boost your energy levels.

The Stress Biology

When you are stressed your hypothalamus will mediate your body's response. The instinctive reaction will be to either run away the circumstances. Ideally, as an evolved human, you'd do the latter. However, stress tends to activate the instinct for survival and self-preservation, which drives you to protect yourself from frightening situations. Keep in mind that many of the human instinctive responses serve to protect us from grave physical danger.

Evolved humans face fewer direct, life-threatening situations, and a lot more mentally threatening situations. For example, when you think about paying your bills, you create a threatening situation in your mind by fearing that your electricity might get shut down. Your brain identifies this thought as threatening and responds accordingly. You are not in a life-threatening situation, but your body may react as if you were.

After the stressful event, situation, or thought passes, the stress hormones, such as noradrenaline, adrenaline, and cortisol, are released into your bloodstream. After an episode of stress passes your body will produce cortisol, which will spike your hunger and desire to eat. After a hypothetically dangerous situation, your body responded as if you had run away, and the innate need to compensate for the energy that has been spent activates. You now have to compensate for the energy that you spent when you were under stress by eating. When your stress is chronic, your body continues to secrete cortisol, which further stimulates your appetite.

A strong appetite after a stressful episode happens as your body's effort to return to balance. However, these efforts will be efficient only temporarily if you experience chronic stress and the constant cortisol response.

Stress eating is the main underlying factor in emotional eating, causing both physiological and emotional responses inside your body. It is one of the strongest emotions, that requires strong coping and management skills to recover from. If you feel like you could be eating out of stress, there are numerous things you can do to alleviate this habit.

There are many triggers for stress eating, such as boredom, routines, tiredness, and fatigue, as well as social influences. Boredom and routines can easily drive stress even if you are not overworking yourself. If you are used to a high-stress lifestyle, having nothing to do can in return cause even more anxiety because you're feeling like you are wasting time. You are feeling a sense of urgency to find something productive to do. Simultaneously, you are chronically overtired and unable to do anything productive. As a result, you are again stressed out, even if you're not doing anything stressful or exhausting. This is consuming your emotional and mental energy.

How to Overcome Stress-Eating

With stress-eating, you are eating for two reasons. The first reason is to calm yourself down, and the second reason is to recover from the loss of energy that happened during the stressful episode. Either way, using this book, you can find some coping strategies to address your stress instead of ignoring it. Here are the steps to recover from stress-eating:

- The first step to prevent stress eating is to learn how to recognize your triggers. To do this, keep a journal and note situations when you feel like you want to eat for other reasons than being physically hungry.

- Next, you want to track your behaviors. This will give you insight into your eating habits. When tracking your hunger or eating behaviors. Include the intensity and the fluctuations of your hunger. You can rate them on a scale of 1 to 10, to compare the intensity of different triggers.

- Also, note the particular activity that you are doing, and whether it is, in any way, unpleasant or annoying.

- Write down the descriptions of feeling physical sensations, and thoughts that come into your mind.

- Start thinking about the ways you can calm yourself without food. Think about other activities that calm you down that you can do instead of eating. Can you listen to music, meditate, read a book, or do yoga? Can you make certain lifestyle changes that will allow more time for rest? If your problem seems to be too difficult to handle on your own, you can always talk to a therapist.

Stress eating can also have a lot to do with your early childhood development. If your parents used food to calm you down instead of teaching you how to process your emotions, you might have learned that the best way to be calm in adult life is by eating.

Another reason that you might be stress-eating is that you have difficulty acknowledging your own feelings. When you have negative feelings, you want to remove or destroy them. This can leave lead to unhealthy behaviors because feelings don't go away when we want them to. You can suppress them, but they will reappear sooner or later.

So, what can you do to stop this? The solution is to break the cycle, discover your personal stress triggers, and find the best ways to cope. You will do this by listing the current influences that are making you feel stressed out. You can do this by sectioning different areas of your life, or by laying out only the most important influences. Here's a small task list to help you out:

- Write down all of the symptoms of stress that you are currently experiencing.

- Sort them by physical, emotional, and psychological.

- After this, it is time to rediscover the ways in which you were using food to cope with stress.

- List the foods that you enjoy eating while you are under stress. Note the amount of food you are eating, and how you feel before and after eating it.

- What do you hope to gain by eating in a stressful situation?

Creating this list of personal insights is a good way for you to figure out how your mind and body choose to cope with stress.

Value Your Sleep

To reduce your chances of eating out of tiredness, it will be convenient for you to get into a good sleeping schedule. You can do this by paying better attention so that you get into bed on time and wake up on time in the morning. If that looks difficult, you can use sleep medication, mindfulness, herbal medicine, therapy, or any other method to regain healthy sleep.

Stress has a lot to do with eating disorders and unhealthy eating behaviors. It becomes a mechanism for you to avoid confrontation with inner demons. With emotional eating, you are regulating the feeling of stress using food, because you believe that you are unable to cope with them otherwise.

Manage Stress Responses

Chronic stress can come in a way of solving your own weight issues and getting better. Stress can wear you down emotionally, spiritually, and physically. Whenever you face the circumstances or the demands that feel overbearing, you will respond with stress. To learn how to cope with stress, you will have to learn how to manage your responses to it. You will start by increasing your awareness of what's going on inside your mind and body. However, the way for you to learn to cope with stress isn't just to change the circumstances, but to also adjust your reaction. When you are avoiding stress, you aren't learning to become mentally resilient. Instead, you are avoiding addressing the true issues by removing the triggers.

Chapter 3: Emotional Eating, Emotional Blocks, and Early Attachment

Originating in early childhood, an attachment style is a form in which you are connected to your primary caregivers. If your attachment style was secure, you've learned that the world is a safe place, in which you are free to explore, and you'll have a safe base to return in the moments when you become lonely or frightened. For a child to form a secure attachment, it is necessary for the caregiver to be attentive, considerate, accepting, and responsive to the child's emotional cues.

It's not uncommon for caregivers to not validate the child's feelings. Depending on how equipped the caregiver is to respond to the child's needs, they might perceive crying, fear, and anger as signs of being spoiled or weak, and they may decide to ignore and punish the expressions of these feelings as a way to 'raise a child well'. While the intention behind this might be good, the results can be detrimental to the mind of a child.

Emotional Blocks And Why They Trigger Emotional Eating

When your emotions are unvalidated in your family, this can lead to problems with emotional regulation, resulting in future eating disorders. If you learned that it is not acceptable to express your emotions, you may have learned to block your feelings through eating. When your feelings were invalidated, and the focus was on control and achievement, and particularly in combination with chronic stress, you were denied the right to cope in a healthy way, and learn from your experiences. This caused you to 'block' certain emotions, deeming them too strong or dangerous to feel and acknowledge their existence.

If you were constantly criticized, invalidated, or abused, you've learned that it is wrong or unsafe for you to express your own feelings. Your emotional needs were not met. This could happen in numerous situations, from not being comforted when crying, to being criticized whenever you rebelled against the caregivers' authority. This might explain why you have problems regulating emotions, and why there are so many emotional blockages present in your mind. Removing these emotional blocks will help you learn how to regulate your own feelings.

How to Overcome Emotional Blocks

To discover and remove emotional blocks, it is best to choose to confront traumatizing events in a mindful fashion. You may choose to do it alone, with a pen and a piece of paper, or, if the past trauma is severe, do it with the help of a therapist. Here are the questions to answer in order to remove emotional blockages:

- Do you remember experiencing intense emotional and physical trauma?

- What do you remember about the situation?

- To track your thoughts, create different columns that will serve to describe the situation (circumstances, events, the setting), the thoughts that were going through your mind, the feelings associated with them, and the physical sensations that these feelings created.

When you've broken down the traumatizing events into the sequences of thoughts, feelings, and sensations, take some time to review and understand how these recollections related to your adult behaviors. Going back to the most traumatizing events from your past might feel unbearably sad or scary. Be open and accepting of your feelings, understanding that, while difficult, this process will help you overcome the pain that was with you all throughout your life. By facing your feelings, you will be able to learn from them and grow. Be open to crying, raging, and expressing these feelings in all ways that aren't threatening to your or others' safety.

Emotional Blocks and Negative Core Beliefs

The negative core beliefs about food are learned for numerous reasons. Due to negative core beliefs, you are living by wrong assumptions. For example, core beliefs that expressing feelings is bad, that fear or sadness makes your week, all boil down to basic needs for safety, love, and trust. If you learned to obtain these in an unhealthy way, it could lead to obesity. When your core beliefs aren't addressed, they aren't allowing you to cope with feelings in a healthy way. When a situation appeals to your negative core belief, it will trigger a strong emotional response. When this happens, you're unable to cope with overwhelming emotions, and you will eat as a way to suppress the sense of endangerment.

Core beliefs form in childhood, during times of transition and emotional development. They become unconscious. Core beliefs will determine the way in which you view yourself, and other people. They will appear in situations that trigger your primal needs for safety, love, validation, and support. As they form as a way of understanding or coping with a certain situation, they will appear when it becomes necessary for you to cope with a certain person or a situation. When these core beliefs aren't being addressed, it can create problems with regulating emotions and stopping the unhealthy behaviors. If you are experiencing problems with eating, you may also carry numerous negative core beliefs, that you only know how to cope with using food.

Feeling like you don't belong, or that there is no one you can count on, that people will take advantage of you, that something is wrong with you, that you are unlovable, that you're born to be unsuccessful, that you're incompetent, that you don't have any direction, or that you are a failure, maybe behind your problems with emotional eating.

If you came from an overly permissive family, you may believe that you should be able to do whatever you want, or you may feel like you have trouble controlling your impulses. If you're taught to put your needs aside, you may feel guilty if you put your own needs before the needs of others. You may feel like your feelings will harm others, and that it won't be good enough, whatever you do. You may also fear that you will hurt others with your feelings, or that you should be punished if you don't meet your own expectations.

When an event or a situation triggers your negative core belief, you will experience the same sensations that you have felt when the belief was formed. It will also trigger the same thoughts and judgments. For example, you may replicate the same exact childhood trauma by being with a partner who is similar to the abuser. This can happen if you are unconsciously trying to win over the abusive, or emotionally unavailable person with love. On the other hand, you may rebel against the belief and be obsessive in doing the exact opposite of what the belief is telling you to do.

Avoidance is another way in which people often cope with negative core beliefs. For example, believing that you are unlovable may lead you to avoid connecting with people both in terms of friendly and romantic relationships. As a result, you might only allow yourself to have a strong relationship with food. As people pick up on your unconscious core beliefs and act according to them, the response that you will be getting will match your core belief. This will, in return, enforce your belief that food is the only source of love, companionship, and pleasure that is available to you.

Whenever you experience an intense feeling of fear, shame, or guilt, you can count on an irrational, negative assumption being behind it. This should be a positive sign that whatever you're feeling, while hurtful, is also inaccurate. Here's how to identify core beliefs that apply to your relationship with food:

- Think about why you are struggling with eating.

- Think about the things that would be missing out from your life if it wasn't replaced by eating.

- Write down what would your greatest fears be.

Now that you are aware of your fears, write down your thoughts until you reach a primal need. Most often, it will be a need for attention, love, acceptance, validation, attention, or companionship. These are the most common core beliefs behind emotional eating:

- 'It doesn't matter how I feel,'

- 'I am better than other people and I deserve something that I don't have,'

- 'I'm stupid/a failure,'

- 'I'm incompetent,'

- 'No one will love me if they know who I am,'

- 'I don't belong,'

- 'People take advantage of me,'

- 'I can't rely on other people,' etc.

- After that, write down the core belief that relates to food. This is the belief that comes to your mind while you're eating. This belief is a guide for you to address the overbearing feelings.

- Next, write down how this belief affects different areas of your life. Focus on your work, relationships, both friendly and romantic, the self-image and body image, sense of security and self-worth, and feeling like you belong to a group.

- Next, try to remember what situations or memories from your past life relate to this feeling.

How to Change Negative Core Beliefs

Becoming aware of your beliefs will help you stop being a slave to their influence. The negative core beliefs are shaping your reality, and you feel like those negative assumptions are your reality. To start shaping your reality by more positive core beliefs, the first step is to start changing your perspective. To a certain degree, just becoming aware of the irrational core belief will relieve the underlying stress and anxiety. However, to truly build yourself up, you will have to look into the way in which the core belief affects your life. The same way that it took years, even decades, for this belief to start molding your life, it will take time for you to practice using a balanced belief to create a more positive outlook.

Be patient and mindful throughout the process. Keep in mind that your core beliefs also shape the way in which other people see you. You are sending signals about your core beliefs through verbal and mental statements, but also more subtle, non-verbal signals, like body language, facial expressions, breathing, eye movement, and physiological responses, like sweating.

When recovering from negative core beliefs, be open to acknowledging that the good part of the negative responses from your environment came from the signals you were sending out unwillingly, and trust that this will change when your attitude changes from the inside out.

Exercise Shifting Perspective

Here's how to exercise shifting your perspective and outlook on diet and eating:

- Track down an event that you remember may have caused a negative core belief that, as you revealed, has to do with your eating habits.

- Visualize being in a courtroom.

- Practice arguing that this belief isn't true, by providing factual evidence.

- List the things you would be comfortable doing to challenge this belief daily.

- Honor the reason why the core belief looked true to you, but acknowledge that it no longer serves you and that you are willing to let go of it.

- State the trust you have in yourself to cope with the challenges that might come your way.

- Establish how the core belief served you.

- Become aware of the skills that you now have to cope with the same situation differently.

- Talk to your younger self and acknowledge their pain. Praise them for coping the best way they could in the situation, and state that what happened in the past was not their fault.

- Formulate a new, positive, balanced core belief.

- Keep in mind that overcoming the negative core beliefs isn't a one-time process. It takes practice and repetition to train your mind to pay better attention to the evidence and triggers of a new, positive core belief, instead of focusing on the negative.

Practice Positive Beliefs

- Write down the new, positive, core belief, and list the principles based on that belief that will be guiding your life from now on.

- Remind yourself of these principles every day. Pay attention to signs that you are slipping back into your old patterns, and be prepared to switch to the new, functional patterns.

- To add more emotional meaning to your new, positive, core beliefs, collect items that symbolize them and keep them across your home and in your office.

Chapter 4: Emotional Eating And Emotional Intelligence

Emotional eating and emotional intelligence share a direct connection. Studies have found that people who have underdeveloped emotional intelligence are more vulnerable to emotional eating. Please, keep in mind that having underdeveloped emotional intelligence doesn't mean that you are overall unintelligent. Emotional intelligence develops in early childhood, and it has a lot to do with the type of attachment you have with your primary caregivers. You learned everything you know about life, as well as the skills to cope with negative feelings, from the people that took care of you as an infant. If you didn't have enough love, acceptance, and understanding, and if your main caregivers weren't very emotionally mature themselves, they were unable to teach you how to understand your own sentiments. As a result, your emotional intelligence may not be as refined as it should be in order to live a healthy, fulfilling life. This can happen even if the family that raised you was loving and attentive.

What Is Emotional Intelligence?

Emotional intelligence is the capacity to observe, understand, evaluate, and navigate your own emotional responses (Zysberg,2018). It has a lot to do with the ability to hold yourself accountable for your own feelings, the understanding that your feelings are a result of an inner reaction rather than an exterior influence, as well as the ability to separate the way you feel in a certain situation from the other person's point of view.

Working to develop your emotional intelligence may help you develop an awareness of your thought process, and the way in which your body reacts by creating feelings. As a result, you may be more aware of your eating habits, and the actual thought process behind your appetite.

It has been found that anxiety mediates the connections between the behavioral patterns in emotional eating and emotional intelligence.

What does this mean? When you are ill-equipped to cope with your own feelings, anxiety will appear as a result. For this reason, you may interpret some of the signs that your body is sending as being hungry, when the true need is for coping and acknowledgment.

Emotional intelligence also affects our food choices. There are many reasons why, when you have a choice to have healthy foods instead of fast food, you may go for the unhealthy option. This difference doesn't have a lot to do with your knowledge about the proper diet. The lack of emotional intelligence has to do with the inability to realize that the reason why you suddenly crave sugars and carbs is in your mind, not the gut. Ideally, you'd be able to notice that you crave fast food or sweets when you're in distress. You would go for a cup of tea as a healthy alternative. With underdeveloped emotional intelligence, that doesn't happen. You are unable to understand why you're drawn to unhealthy snacks. You're unable to address the real problem, or at least find a healthier substitute.

The sentiments that are behind your relationship with food need to be addressed, and with lack of the right skills you are either suppressing or misinterpreting them.

What Are the Qualities of Emotionally Intelligent Eaters?

To better understand the need to learn the skills of emotional coping and regulation, it's useful to look into the ways in which people with properly developed emotional intelligence think and act in relation to food, health, and weight loss. An emotionally intelligent eater understands how emotions affect their diet decisions. To them, this process is conscious and they are aware of it. Self-awareness is an important part of emotional intelligence and includes the ability for a person to understand what is happening inside them. If you are an emotionally intelligent eater, you will notice when you are feeling stressed, and that stress causes the sensations that might come off as hunger. Instead of binge eating, an emotionally mature eater is able to take some time and calm down first, after which they'll reflect on whether or not they really need food, and which foods are the best option.

Impulse Control

Emotionally intelligent eaters have their impulses and sudden feelings under control. Instead of reacting impulsively to their emotions, emotionally intelligent eaters are able to take a step back and think about what's going on inside their bodies. Instead of resorting to food, they will take a break, have a short walk outside, or talk to a friend. This way, they have an opportunity to process their experiences and hardships in a healthy way.

Adaptability

Emotionally intelligent eaters easily adapt when they experience unexpected stress or circumstances. They understand that stress can't be avoided and that the best way to cope with it is to calm down, assess the situation, prioritize, regroup, or do whatever it takes to 'get back on track.'

Level-Headedness

Emotionally intelligent eaters are able to stick to their diet (and other) plans, regardless of distractions.

While there's no need for them to be strict or rigid about the way they eat, they will still manage to follow through their schedule and work around obstacles patiently and without tension.

Assertiveness

Emotionally intelligent eaters are good at saying 'no.' To become an emotionally intelligent eater, you will practice your right to say 'no' and refuse to do things for people you're uncomfortable doing, including courtesy eating. This applies to situations when you are offered foods, and you only eat to avoid refusing, or offending other people. Emotional eaters often eat when they don't need to because they feel uncomfortable rejecting an offer. In addition, they also have a hard time saying 'no' to doing things they don't want to do or eat as a result of suppressing the stress that the decision causes them.

Flexibility

Emotionally intelligent eaters persist in doing their tasks and meeting goals regardless of obstacles. They won't be easily upset if unpredictable circumstances disrupt their schedule. Rather than responding with stress, panic, confusion, or anger, emotionally intelligent eaters are flexible. They think about ways to overcome obstacles, instead of stressing over disruptions When it comes to weight loss, emotionally intelligent eaters look at the big picture and are most likely to maintain the weight loss in the long run. They focus less on keeping their diet and exercise schedule perfect, and more on long-term progress.

Compassion

Emotionally intelligent eaters treat others and their weight issues with compassion. They are less likely to judge those who are overweight and struggle with weight loss. They think of themselves in a more positive manner, and are, accordingly, more compassionate to others as a result. Emotionally intelligent eaters are aware that everyone struggles from time to time, and that not everyone is able to stay persistent and power through obstacles. They treat people who are in trouble with kindness and understanding.

Respectful Agility

Emotionally intelligent eaters are very good at balancing their needs with those of others. They are skillful in rejecting foods in a way that is respectful and appreciative of others. They won't get upset if food is offered to them, and they won't feel anxious about rejecting the food in a respectful way. They will find ways to be a part of the group, even when they're choosing not to eat, or choosing more diet-friendly options.

How To Enhance Emotional Intelligence

You can work on advancing your emotional skills to become better in regulating your emotions and eating habits. Boosting emotional intelligence, accompanied by an improvement of eating habits, can have long-term positive effects on your well-being. The first thing you need to do is understand that your feelings affect your body in a physical way. Every feeling you feel will have a physical impact on your heart rate and the way you feel on the inside.

Give Your Food the Right Meaning

Becoming an emotionally intelligent eater means focusing not only on the food you eat but also on the way you eat. It means understanding that the food has a bigger impact on your body than just making you feel full. Food is the source of mental and emotional satisfaction. But, in order to boost your emotional intelligence in relation to food, you need to look into the right ways to find satisfaction in eating. Researching for the most health-beneficial foods, making sure that you are enjoying the process of preparing food, making your meals look nice, and understanding the way in which all of this affects your inner being is the first step to boosting your emotional intelligence with eating.

Look Inside

Emotionally intelligent eaters understand that recovering from emotional eating is more about looking inside, and altering your lifestyle, then simply changing the way you eat. To boost your emotional intelligence about food, be constantly aware of the triggers, thoughts, beliefs, and assumptions that lie behind the cravings. This may take a lot of work at first, but it will pay off in the long run.

Be Accountable

Accountability is an important part of emotional intelligence. It means understanding that you have control over your thoughts and actions and that they don't control you. Becoming more emotionally intelligent means understanding that you are making a conscious choice to eat, and what to eat. The same way, making a commitment to yourself not to blame the food, your family, or anyone else for your current eating situation, means acknowledging that the improvement is your responsibility.

In this chapter, you learned the impact that emotional intelligence has on emotional eating. Now that you know why you're having trouble understanding the way you feel, and what you can do to improve, it's time to learn how to stop ignoring your own emotional needs and voice them to relieve inner tension and find the support that you deserve.

Chapter 5: How to Voice Your Needs and Stop Suppressing

Learning how to voice your needs might be challenging if you're used to staying quiet and keeping to yourself. Still, realizing that you are overeating to block the feelings you aren't acknowledging, should make you wonder if you are expressing yourself enough. You may be insufficiently vocal in speaking out when you are hurt, scared, angry, and in need for compassion. Below this silence lies many dysfunctional beliefs, such as:

- Speaking up will disturb, hurt, or offend those closest to you;

- Admitting being angry, sad, or scared, means that you are weak or incompetent;

- No one will understand the way you feel;

- If you speak your mind, people will think that you are selfish/spoiled/irrational, etc.;

- If you open up about your feelings, the person won't validate them, and that will only hurt you more; and

- There's no point in voicing your needs. They don't matter, and no one will listen anyways;

If you shy away from voicing your needs out of fear that you will be misunderstood, judged, or rejected, work on acknowledging your own, unconditional right to understanding and compassion. Being open to and understanding someone's feelings doesn't cost or hurt anyone, so there's no rational excuse to deny compassion. Even if it is true that a specific thing you are yearning for is unavailable, you benefit from taking back your right to be heard, acknowledged, and respected.

Being unwilling to voice your needs may also compromise your relationships, both familial and romantic. Without speaking out on the things that hurt you and asking for love when you need it, those closest to you don't get the opportunity to help. If your requests for validation, compassion, and understanding remain ignored, you may want to rethink your relationships. As an adult, you're in no way obliged to have a relationship with anyone. A one-sided relationship, in which you are the one who doesn't get any respect or acknowledgment, doesn't serve you.

Be Aware Of Negative Thoughts

Negative self-directed talk, both conscious and unconscious, is a learned behavior that relates to suppressing feelings due to negative self-image. It is a learned thought pattern that you've adopted in early childhood, which can put you in a state of 'emotional fog.' Because negative self-talk is profoundly scary and hurtful, it will cause a lot of emotional ambivalence. Emotional ambivalence means that you are facing a lot of conflicting emotions at once, and it is a difficult state to be in. On the one side, there's the negative self-talk, but on the other, there are your inborn needs for love, support, acceptance, as well as the 'rebellion' to these thoughts. Your unconscious negative self-talk hurts you emotionally, and you are simultaneously defending against it. This creates emotional conflicts that feel deeply disturbing, and you may find overeating to be the only way to quiet these loud, conflicting feelings and thoughts. In this case, food is the way to clear your mind and ground yourself, but it is a bad way.

You can get into a state of an emotional fog if your relationships were chronically stressful for a long time. In this situation, you are feeling an overwhelming number of conflicting emotions that are draining you both physically and mentally. This can happen if you've had an insecure attachment with your primary caregivers. Insecure attachment makes you more easily alerted, and your insecurities are more easily triggered.

Example

You can see a happy couple on the street, feel unbearable hunger, and head straight to the fast-food stand. On your way there, you are feeling stressed, nervous, sad, and angry. Why is this happening? Better yet, what is happening inside you? Here's the explanation:

- Seeing the happy couple at first made you happy because you believe in love;

- Feeling the belief in love triggered your core belief that you're unworthy of love;

- At the same time, this core belief reminded you of your need to be loved and all the ways in which that is currently not happening for you;

- The inner conflict is created. You have conflicting beliefs of love and your unworthiness of love, and at the same time a strong need for love.

- All of this happening in a split-second. Your mind is unable to process all of these intense thoughts, and a strong emotional response is triggered. You are anxious, and your stomach is upset;

- You only know to calm yourself with food. Thinking about the current situation isn't something you learned. As the sensations feel overwhelming, you instinctively grab the first thing that helps you calm down, which is an over-sized portion of fast food.

- You are eating, and starting to calm down. You realize that you ate all of this food without a need to eat. Now, you feel ashamed of your own behavior, and your emotional conflict is still there, only temporarily alleviated. You will most likely feel sad and depressed for a while, anywhere between a couple of hours to a couple of days.

When you're in a state of emotional fog, you are experiencing the lack of emotional regulation on a very organic level. Being aware of the attachment styles that have shaped your childhood and adult relationships will enable you to form a mechanism for healthy coping.

Replace Negative With Positive Thoughts

While you can't go back in time and secure yourself a healthy upbringing, now as an adult, you are able to give yourself the teaching and support that is necessary to learn how to cope in healthy, functional ways. Some of the lessons to teach yourself are:

- To bring awareness to alerting, 'red flag,' thoughts and feelings with acceptance and understanding; ('This couple reminds me that I want love and I don't have it.' 'I feel unworthy of love, but I need it, and this makes me sad.')

- To shed light on how your feelings affect your actions; ('I feel like I want to eat now, but if I do, it won't help. It will only make me feel worse. I want to find other ways to calm down.')

- To find healthy ways to cope with overwhelming feelings, such as:

    o Calm yourself down;

    o Replace negative with balanced, rational self-talk; and

    o Talk to yourself until you're more convinced into the rational point of view rather than self-negative ideas;

Example

'While this situation makes me sad, I choose to honor and accept my pain. Yes, I haven't been loved and cared for enough. But that doesn't mean I'm unworthy of love. There's hope for me to find a good, loving companion. There's no reason for me not to find love. It may be a rocky road, and I might look for love in the wrong places. But I choose to be with someone who loves and respects me, and I choose to respect myself while looking for love.'

- To bring awareness to the necessity of moving on with daily activities; ('I feel hurt now, but I will proceed with my normal schedule. I don't have to stop this feeling to have a good, productive day').

- Balancing out the need to vent with the need to stay level-headed; ('While I acknowledge my pain, I will proceed with the things I planned to do. I will go to work, and see my friend afterwards. When the time seems right, I may cry or talk about my experience with those who are able to understand.')

- Finding ways to proceed with normal daily activities while acknowledging the feeling of distress with:

    - Accepting, positive self-talk; ('I am a wonderful person who is worthy of love. It may not have been my experience, but I have the power to make it my experience and be loved the way I deserve to be loved.')

    - Understanding that you don't need to 'pause' your life until you feel good again; (*While I feel sad, I won't let it overpower me.*)

    - Measuring the right pace for yourself while you are feeling distressed: To what degree will you reduce activities to give yourself space to hurt and heal, without compromising your own work and relationships? To what degree will you try to 'power through' difficult situations without self-neglect, burning out, or suppressing your feelings?

To get out of the emotional fog and step into a healthy place of emotional regulation, it is essential for you to understand that there's no point in trying to erase or replace the negatives (feelings, events, memories, circumstances). To you, it might look like the people around you all come from a stable background and are always emotionally balanced and fulfilled. Are you sure that the couple from the example above are happy? Perhaps, they've held each other to comfort one another because one of them is ill. You don't know if the couple maybe lost a child, or there's adultery in the relationship, or perhaps even abuse. Or they just as well might be as happy as they seem. But, none any of that means that you won't be able to be happy.

The way to find an emotional balance, while acknowledging your negative thoughts, is to understand that the negatives in life can't and shouldn't be erased or replaced. There is nothing abnormal about feeling down, as long as you are able to understand that feeling down doesn't mean allowing yourself to fall down. In terms of emotional eating, your goal isn't to stop or re-train yourself to feel only positive to avoid overeating. Instead, your goal is preventing the negatives from being the reason you eat. It is the behavior, the response, that you will be working to change, not yourself or your emotions.

Rely On Support To Feel Hopeful

Having a support system while working to recover from emotional eating will help you overcome the emotional blocks that are holding you down. Learning how to open up to those who are close to you and care about you will help you to stop suppressing feelings, and open up to the idea of self-compassion and self-validation. The following members of your closest community will help you recover and regain hope:

Friends And Family

While some of the issues that caused your eating problem may root in the childhood and the way in which you were brought up, that doesn't mean that your family is a bad influence to stay away from. On the contrary. You can use the adult relationships that you have with your family members to be emotionally mature, and overcome the burdens that you've been carrying on your back. The role of your familiar circle isn't just to support you through weight loss. You can share your insights with them, and reach out to voice your deepest needs, forgive, and heal from old trauma.

Your Therapist

As you learned while reading this book, the process of building yourself up to overcome emotional eating can be liberating, but also confusing and emotionally hurtful. While delving into your deepest fears and painful memories, you will use the guidance of a trained, qualified expert. A therapist will guide you to reach the right conclusions, preventing further irrational assumptions. If emotional eating has to do with traumatic experiences or loss, the intensity of recalling these events might be severe. You may experience panic, anxiety attacks, or thoughts of self-harming. For this reason, it is smart to have someone by your side who is professionally trained for mental and emotional support. Your therapist will show you how to cope with intense pain, fear, and anxiety, and they will also teach you how to change your relationship with food on a more personal level, tailored to your unique background and life experiences.

Your Doctor

Emotional eating, particularly combined with obesity, could have damaged your health. Your doctor will help you include all dietary considerations into your meal plan and schedule. They will tell you how to use food to heal your body instead of damaging it.

Your doctor will also give instructions on the right foods and portion sizes, so that you stay happy and fulfilled while dieting.

Chapter 6: Emotional Eating, Resistance to Diet, and Unconscious Eating

Eating is over-learned behavior. This means that most people eat as a part of their daily lives, without much thought of what to eat. This chapter will focus on the reasons why you are harboring such strong resistance to a healthy diet. In this chapter, you will learn what refusing to eat healthily has to do with refusing to acknowledge your own sentiments, and the profound insecurities that 'pull the strings' of your eating decisions (Ross, 2016).

What is Unconscious Eating?

Automatic eating is an unconscious behavior that begins without intention to eat, carries on without control, and goes on with very little effort to prevent the behavior. Just being near the food can become enough of a trigger to some people. Mindfulness can help you bring awareness to eating, and shed light on the background of your cravings. This way, you will become more successful in regulating your eating habits and weight.

When you are eating on impulse, eating becomes a fast reaction to a trigger without considering the negative consequences. When you're impulsive about eating, you are having trouble controlling your eating behaviors, and you become powerless to delay the gratification of your urges. Mindfulness can help you reduce these impulsive behaviors and get profound insight into what happens inside your mind when you get a sudden urge to eat.

On the behavioral side of emotional eating, the problem is starting to eat without paying attention. You may be eating on auto-pilot, completely unaware that you are doing it. One of the ways to stop this is to become a mindful eater. If eating is an automatic process for you, ending this habit means learning how to eat consciously, with focus and appreciation.

Overcome Unconscious With Mindful Eating

Mindful eating can help you manage your weight and stop unconscious eating. Mindful eating has become popular as a way of coping with eating behaviors and promoting weight loss. Research has found that mindful meditation that focuses on eating may help promote healthier eating behaviors and regulate weight.

What Is Mindful Eating?

To better explain how mindfulness can help you overcome emotional eating, let's define mindfulness first. You can think of mindfulness as a state of awareness that happens when you purposefully direct your attention to the present moment. You can also think about mindfulness as a way to use awareness for self-regulation and to intentionally focus your attention on a certain aspect of your health, life, or behavior.

Mindfulness is, most often, practiced through meditation and self-reflection. This helps you divert your attention from food, dieting, and exercise, which are only the superficial aspects of healing, to your inner being, its fears and needs.

Being mindful also challenges you to stop being judgmental of your thoughts and feelings. Instead, you are to be open and compassionate when confronting fears, anger, and personal issues. Being mindful can help you reduce automatic eating, as well as the responses to emotional triggers. Both of these behaviors lead to eating when you don't need to, and choosing less healthy foods.

How to Practice Mindful Eating

Emotional eating can appear as a result of using food to cope with overwhelming sensations. It becomes a tool for you to suppress negative feelings and thoughts. It is a form of avoidance that temporarily relieves negative thoughts and feelings. Without processing those thoughts and feelings, they will inevitably come back, triggering yet another emotional eating episode. When this becomes a learned pattern, you will have more frequent episodes as a result of suppressing emotions.

The weight gain, as well as a decay of overall health and mental wellbeing, come as a result of this long-term pattern. To become mindful about your automatic eating habits, you can choose to stop and analyze the thoughts that are going through your mind when you feel a sudden urge to eat. You can think back to the situation and reflect on the circumstances, words being said to you, and thoughts that resulted from these circumstances. You can write down these thoughts and the way that they made you feel. As you delve into your emotional issues, the food cravings should reduce. By repeating this process over time, you will train your mind to become more aware of the triggers, and you'll become better at noticing the true causes of the sudden, unbearable appetite.

Learning the right techniques of mindful meditation is neither fast nor easy. It will require training and guidance by qualified experts, but the results will, by far, be worthy of the investment. There are two simple ways in which you can introduce mindfulness into your eating habits:

Meditation

Meditation isn't easy to learn, but it can help you become more aware of thoughts and feelings you are associating with food.

While effective meditation requires assistance from a trained expert, learning the skill will help you become more aware of the sensations that your thoughts and feelings trigger within your body, that relate to appetite.

Conscious Eating

Mindful eating requires you to be slow, patient, respectful, grateful, and appreciative of your food. When eating, you should take your time to savor the flavors and textures, thinking about the health impact that these foods will have on your body. While eating, you may focus on feeling grateful for these foods. You can also focus on the pleasant sensations that these foods are creating in different parts of your body, such as tongue, mouth, throat, and stomach. During and after eating, you can focus on the ways in which these foods are benefitting your body and health, as well as making you happy. Mindful eating requires you to remove any distractions, such as your phone or laptop, to fully focus on the foods that you are eating.

How Unconscious Eating and Emotional Blocks Cause Emotional Eating

Identifying and acknowledging your own feelings is often easier done for others than within ourselves. You have learned to pay attention to others' emotions, but not your own. The problem with emotional eating is that you are restraining from acknowledging your own emotions. This could have happened for numerous reasons. You may not have been thought to do it, or you might have learned that sadness, fear, or insecurity, are a sign of weakness. Even happiness, in some families, can be seen as irresponsibility, and you may eat to punish yourself for feeling happy.

The Inability to Communicate Feelings

If you were raised in a way to think that being emotional means being weak, you are lacking the skills to identify the emotions you are feeling. Here's how you can learn to better identify your own feelings:

- List situations in which you feel particular emotions.

- Write down physical sensations that you feel across the different parts of your body.

- What about your body language? What are you doing with your arms and legs?

- What about facial expressions? Are you clenching your jaw, cringing, or opening your eyes wider?

- Ask yourself what you are feeling. You can choose whichever way works for you to record your findings, like journaling or recording.

Not being able to understand the cues of your body is often behind emotional eating. It is the lack of ability to communicate emotions through verbal and non-verbal signals, both with yourself and with others. As you haven't learned to communicate your feelings to other people, you may have become unable to communicate them to yourself. Furthermore, expressing the feelings you feel are a sign of weakness can cause intense stress or guilt.

Emotional Suppression

Knowing the reason why you are suppressing feelings will help you discover the wrong beliefs you carry about communicating emotions. Here's how to discover the reasons behind suppression and overcome it once and for all:

- Write down how and why do you feel like expressing certain feelings is wrong.

- Write down what would have changed for you if you didn't think it was wrong.

- Write down how you perceive food relates to relieving particular emotions.

- Write down the rules about feelings that you've learned, such as: 'Don't trust your emotions,' 'Keep your emotions to yourself,' 'You don't have the right to be angry, sad, scared, or even happy.'

The 'rules' you've been taught to follow when regulating feelings are acting unconsciously and stirring the way in which you understand inner sensations. Knowing exactly how you've been taught to treat yourself when angry, scared, or insecure, will help you understand why you're choosing to escape these feelings.

Doing the above-mentioned exercise will help you re-experience and acknowledge the feelings that you wanted to express but somehow weren't allowed to.

Projecting Feelings Onto Others to Avoid Facing Them

Emotional eating may also be about the desire to swallow down the feelings instead of facing and coping with past hurt or fear. Holding on to the judgment of others that have hurt you only hurts you further, preventing you from living in the present time. In this sense, you are eating to cope with being hurt by others, but never healing from it. You may have learned this behavior if you were offered snacks to calm down, instead of support, consolation, and the right advice to process your feelings.

Feeling Ashamed of Your Own Feelings

Not everyone learns to accept their feelings as a child. Your caregivers might have taught you that crying means being weak, or that you are being a bad person when you get angry. All of these early lessons might have taught you to feel ashamed of expressing your feelings. As a result, you never learned to regulate them and cope with them in a healthy way. Once you learn to regulate emotions, you will no longer have to use food as a way to regain a sense of peace and safety.

Emotional overeaters have trouble managing their emotions. If you have difficulty acknowledging your feelings, you will eat in response to emotional cues. If you are unconsciously ashamed of your feelings, eating might be a way for you to try to change them. This often results in binge-eating, which, in return, causes you to feel even more shame, guilt, and anger with yourself.

Emotional Eating, Isolation, and Rejecting Support

Shutting yourself out from the love and support of others is perhaps the most difficult part about emotional eating. You may be struggling with low self-esteem, stress, and sadness, but still putting on a brave face for everyone around you. While keeping your troubles to yourself shelters you from the feeling of shame, and relieves your fear of being judged, it does a disservice to your health and recovery.

Why Opening Up Is Important

Opening up about your struggles with emotional eating will empower you in many ways. You will acknowledge your own pain and suffering, and let those around you know that you're not as tough as you look. In return, your loved ones will become aware of your need for love and support. Perhaps, they were willing to support you all along, but didn't know you needed their help. In a way, putting on a brave face shelters your loved ones from hurt, but on the other hand, it distances you from them. By staying closed, you are further isolating yourself from the people who can help you the most.

Aside from friends and family, you may be avoiding asking for help from experts. Doctors, psychologists, fitness trainers, and dieticians, are all there to help people just like you. You may be ashamed of your thoughts, fears, habits, or weight. However, keep in mind that the experts who can help you didn't obtain their qualifications to work with people with no issues. On the contrary, they've built their careers around supporting people who have troubles, and feel like they have no one to talk to. Many fitness trainers come from a place of being overweight themselves, doctors decide to pursue medicine because someone close to them was ill, and psychologists choose to help people with emotional struggles because they, or someone close to them, suffered as well.

While you may hesitate to talk about your problems because you feel ashamed, you are forgetting that, expert or not, most people have dealt with seemingly unsolvable problems at one point of their lives. Powering through the feeling of shame, guilt, and powerlessness might not feel good at the moment, but you'll benefit in many ways as you work to heal. For example:

- Learning that many people face similar problems as you;

- Learning that people appreciate the qualities of your personality that you may not be aware of; and

- Learning that people care about you more than you think they do.

If you feel uncomfortable opening up to the people who know you personally, you can always find a support group, either online or offline, that serves people who struggle with emotional eating find help and comfort.

Chapter 7: Learn How to Distinguish the Emotional from Physical Hunger

In order to stop unconscious eating, and bringing more awareness into your eating patterns, you should learn to distinguish physical from emotional hunger. To help you learn how to do this, this chapter will explain the difference in physical sensations, as well as suggest the right ways for you to track the cues of your body to know whether or not you're actually hungry (Konttinen et. al., 2010).

Learn The Difference Between Emotional and Physical Hunger

There are numerous ways for you to learn how to differentiate emotional from physical hunger. Here's how you'll know if your appetite is coming from your stomach, or your mind:

- Think about how the feeling of hunger came to be. If the hunger came quickly and suddenly, it's most likely emotional. Physical hunger starts increasing gradually. It only becomes unbearable if you haven't eaten for an entire day.

- Are you craving specific food? If you need a specific type of food when you are feeling hungry, it is probably due to emotional reasons. During physical hunger, you would feel satisfied eating any type of food, and you wouldn't crave specifically junk-food.

- Are you eating in a mindless way? If you catch yourself eating without even noticing it, it might be emotional hunger and not physical.

- Are there physical symptoms of hunger? If you are physically hungry, your stomach will growl and you'll feel an increase of saliva in your mouth, while emotional hunger starts when you think about food.

- Are you experiencing guilt or shame for eating? Eating out of physical hunger will make you feel satisfied, while eating out of emotional hunger will make you feel ashamed.

Learn to Track Feelings And Physical Sensations to Distinguish Emotional from Physical Hunger

One of the ways for you to learn to distinguish the real from emotional appetite is to trace the body sensations and compare those that appear when you are hungry, and those that appear when you're distressed. Here's how to do it:

- Note the sensations inside your body that occur when you are physically hungry. Pay attention to:

    - The sensations in your stomach;

    - The sensations in your mouth and throat;

    - The changes in these sensations when you are thinking about food; and

    - How the sensations change after you eat;

- Note the sensations inside your body when you feel distressed, such as:

    - The sensations inside your stomach;

    - The sensations in your throat and mouth;

    - Your breathing;

    - How these sensations change when you think about food?

    - How these sensations change when you think about the disturbing situation or event?

    - How do you feel while you're eating? How do the physical sensations change? and

- How do you feel after eating?

Read these observations, and compare them to find the subtle differences in the way your body acts when you are physically hungry, and when you're distressed. This way, you'll learn how to distinguish the two. Soon, you will be able to tell when you are truly hungry, which will help you overcome habitual and stress-eating.

Chapter 8: Learn How To Develop Healthy Coping Mechanisms

Replacing habitual eating with facing, processing, and coping, is crucial to recover from emotional eating. This chapter will help you understand why you've become detached from your inner self, and why have you learned that the best way to cope is to suppress. This process doesn't happen overnight. In this chapter, we will address the causes of emotional detachment that appear in early childhood (Ross, 2016). By looking into the possible reasons why you started to avoid acknowledging your feelings, you will understand where the sudden appetite comes from. Furthermore, this chapter will help you regain a steady, profound relationship with your inner voice. By listening to that inner voice, you will become aware of your true feelings, and with the right guidance, you will be able to cope with your feelings in a healthy way (Evers et. al., 2010).

Listen To Your Inner Voice

Learning how to identify your feelings, and understanding the way in which they affect your appetite, will help replace emotional eating with healthy coping mechanisms.

The emotional experiences you had in the early childhood may trigger in certain situations. They can become a driving force behind your eating. If you haven't learned how to cope with feelings in a healthy way, you may want to escape being overwhelmed by eating.

Rather than suppressing, your goal should be to learn how to identify, express, and regulate emotions. Emotional regulation means that you are able to cope with your feelings in a healthy, functional way. But, how to do that? If you have trouble even acknowledging the way you truly feel, how are you to process?

To answer these questions, keep in mind that your emotions are caused by your thoughts. A thought causes emotion and not the other way around. When you've discovered which exact feeling cause the overwhelming appetite, you can proceed to discover which thoughts have caused this emotion.

When you become aware of triggering thoughts, you can proceed to analyze which assumptions and beliefs lie behind them.

Understand The Signals Of Your Body

Refusing to feel overwhelming emotions creates emotional blocks and leads to overeating. To overcome this, you can practice studying your body image in a mindful way. The goal is to stir your focus from eating and move it inwards, towards listening and acknowledging the sensations that are coming from your body.

Lack of basic care and insufficient self-care in your adult life may cause you to neglect yourself. If you haven't had a good relationship with your caregiver, it resulted in the lack of ability to connect your body, feel it's natural needs, and be open to responding to them. Early attachment identification is important to move towards healing and finding your authentic self. You can identify your attachment style by talking to your therapist or taking an online test.

Dissatisfaction with your body may cause you to disconnect from body sensations, which are a way for your body to communicate its needs with you. You may check your body regularly, but avoid acknowledging the sensations of your body. While you obsess over your weight and shape, you will avoid looking at your body itself and the way it feels.

Overcome Body Detachment With Meditation and Mindfulness

The body image is the picture in your mind that you hold of your own body. If it is negative, you may overeat due to the feeling of shame and guilt. Media can contribute to a negative body image, by creating exaggerated, unrealistic, distorted standards of beauty. Your body also stores many parental influences, such as those of attachment. Your caregivers may have impacted your body image in many ways, from setting the standards of beauty, to teaching you how to 'read' the signals of your body.

How Avoidant Parenting Causes Body Detachment

When your needs were ignored as a child, you will see yourself as an independent person. You will have difficulty bonding with other people, but also with your own body. As you were used to being ignored when in need of affection, you will learn to ignore the warning signs of your body as well. Accordingly, you won't be very insightful about the ways in which your body acts when it's hungry, and the way in which it signals emotional needs. This creates confusion and may result in thinking that you are hungry in situations when you need comforting, rest, company, or love.

Body Detachment and Post Traumatic Stress (PTSD)

If you haven't resolved childhood trauma, your body, and mind may stay frozen in the traumatic moments. When stress or anxiety occur, your childhood trauma will feel like it's happening right now causing you to dissociate. If you haven't acknowledged the feelings surrounding a traumatic event, this process will be unconscious, and you may confuse the feeling of panic with the need to eat. As a result, you will feel stressed and overwhelmed and over-eat to cope.

Discover Core Needs to Overcome Emotional Blocks

As we already mentioned, emotional eating can happen if you are eating to find the satisfaction that you are otherwise denying yourself. One of the ways to stop emotional eating is to look into your deeper needs, and discover what you truly desire to obtain with food.

Discover Core Needs With Mindfulness

You can distinguish true from superficial dietary needs by analyzing your thoughts and feelings. To do this, look into the ways that food is compensating for the lack in your life, versus nourishing and enriching you. To do this, try the following exercises:

- State your values and write them down on a piece of paper.

- Write down how you feel when you live according to your values.

- Write down the ways in which you are satisfied with the way you tend to your values daily and those that you're not satisfied with.

- Look into those areas where you're happy with the way in which you tend to what you value the most in your life. Describe the ways in which you do that in detail.

- Next, look into the areas of your core values that you feel you aren't giving enough attention to, and list the ways in which you want to improve.

With these lists and tasks, you will be more aware of the ways in which you want to nurture your identity through your diet. You can turn to these insights whenever you feel burdened by your eating and weight issues. This will help you shift focus from food onto the ways you can nurture yourself emotionally and spiritually. You can also use these observations to think about the ways in which you want to use food to uplift yourself spiritually, rather than to use it to neglect and avoid fulfilling your spiritual needs.

Anchor to Unveil The Unconscious

Habitual eating that roots in untruthful beliefs, can be changed by working to build a strong bond with your true identity. You will do this by learning the process of anchoring.

Finding your inner anchor means tapping into your intuition and natural instincts that will help you manage the unconscious behaviors and take them in a more positive, healthier direction. When you are detached from your true self (thoughts, feelings, desires), you are unable to interpret the life around you accurately and with enough reasoning. Instead, you go by the superficial, inaccurate assumptions that you've adopted during early childhood. If you're afraid that reaching into the realm of your inner self will result in unreasonable, 'crazy' thoughts, that will somehow harm you, that is yet another irrational, untruthful belief. Much of the 'unreasonable' you've detected by now actually comes from being detached from your true identity, and the refusal to act according to it.

In a detached state, your body and mind will remain stuck in past events, re-living the past pain and trauma. You will respond with eating, unwilling to truly cope and move on from past events. Your health and life will suffer. Rationally, the only way to heal is to find a way to step out of that state and steer your thoughts according to rational, balanced, beliefs.

Finding your anchor means staying in tune with your true self every step of the way. It means being authentic. This way, you will build a healthy, nourishing relationship with food. You will acknowledge your body's need for healthy, nutritious fruits of nature, and you will start to enjoy doing what your body's most innate need is to move, stretch your muscles, circulate your blood, and fill lungs with life-bringing oxygen.

Chapter 9: Emotional Eating and Self Esteem

This chapter will show you just how amazingly complex, and a unique creature you are. Your mind and your stomach are tightly connected. Whole foods fuel your brain, and your brain communicates with your stomach when other channels of communication are unavailable. Everything you do, feel, or think reflects on the way you eat. This includes the way you think and feel about yourself. Your self-esteem largely dictates your relationship with food. Your diet habits are a result of the way in which you've learned to take care of yourself. Ideally, you will love yourself a lot, and want to cherish your body with quality food. If your self-esteem is compromised, you might start to neglect the needs of your body as a way to punish yourself. This chapter will help you understand not only how your self-esteem affects emotional eating, but also what you can do to improve self-image and learn to take good care of yourself.

How Low Self-Esteem Contributes to Emotional Eating

Damaged self-esteem links to emotional eating (Ross,2016). You might be eating to compensate for feeling less worthy, and all of the challenges that you are facing arise from that. Low self-esteem links to the majority of eating disorders as well. As a result of an impaired self-esteem, all of your efforts to establish healthy eating habits might be ineffective long-term. If your idea of recovering from emotional eating is to diet, you are addressing only the smallest part of the problem.

Without working to improve your relationship with yourself, you will be more prone to developing the habit of unconscious eating. Here are some of the ways in which low self-esteem fuels emotional eating:

Crediting Yourself for Failures, but not Successes

At the very root of your self-esteem issues is the habit of denying all of your good sides, successes, and efforts, but highlight your negatives and failures. You are exaggerating the things you are doing wrong, and you're insufficiently aware of the things you are doing right. As a result, you are denying yourself the right to truly enjoy all aspects of your life, making food your only reward, or source of pleasure. With impaired self-esteem, you are denying your own right to be happy and healthy. You think that you don't deserve happiness, or that you didn't work hard enough for it. As a result, you only allow yourself to be happy and satisfied when you are eating.

Feeling Like You Deserve Self-care

When your self-esteem is diminished, you don't feel like you deserve to be well taken care of, both by other people and by yourself. As a result of this belief, you are putting in a lot of effort to take good care of other people but fall into self-neglect. To make the matter worse, as you feel unworthy of love and others' care, you are probably keeping your problem to yourself and avoiding asking for help. Both in terms of emotional eating, as well as other emotional and physical needs, you are avoiding speaking up, and opening up to others' help, love, and kindness. As a result of feeling unworthy of love and care, you neglect yourself to the point when eating enormous amounts of unhealthy foods becomes the only source of pleasure you'll allow yourself.

Feeling Unworthy of Taking the Time for Yourself

In a busy life, valuing oneself enough to set time aside for self-care is a challenge. In terms of eating, you may think of yourself as unworthy of investing the money into good foods, investing the time to make delicious, nutritious meals, and investing the time to eat slowly, with enjoyment and appreciation.

Feeling Unworthy of Healthy Foods

One of the reasons behind making unhealthy food choices is deeming yourself unworthy of healthy food. You may feel like you haven't done or achieved enough in your life to be worthy of a healthy diet, since quality foods tend to be costly. The road to overcoming this belief is working to acknowledge that self-worth is unconditional. There is nothing that you have to achieve, or do, to deserve a healthy diet. Your body needs healthy nutrients, and giving them to yourself doesn't have to be something you deserve. It can be a simple, rational decision, that doesn't have any emotional significance.

Depriving Yourself of Healthy Foods

As a result of self-neglect, you are failing to eat healthy meals on time. As time passes, and your body becomes starved; it is inevitable to over-eat sooner or later. The starvation may drive you to make unhealthy choices, like ordering large amounts of take-out or fast food.

How To Improve Self-Esteem to Overcome Emotional Eating

Improving your self-image will take time, patience, and practice. It can't happen overnight, because you've spent long years of your life training your brain to harbor negative self-beliefs and attitudes towards your own body. Rather than waiting for your body to change for you to like it better, you can focus on making small efforts to feel better right now. Here are a couple of suggestions:

Self-Care

Self-care means giving yourself the right amount of both physical and emotional care. On a physical level, you should focus on powering the body with the right nutrients, to make it strong and healthy. Emotional self-care is done through love, connection, and affection, both with yourself and other people. From a place of emotional eating, your focus should be on nourishment, instead of restriction. When it comes to diet, your thoughts shouldn't be on cutting calories, but replacing them with healthier options instead.

Enjoying Movement

If you're coming from a place of inactivity and a sedentary lifestyle, you won't be able to jump into a rigorous workout routine right away. Your initial steps will be to start to enjoy moving your body. Traditional exercise might be unappealing because you are focusing on the element of hardship and self-punishing for the unhealthy lifestyle. This might ruin your efforts to exercise and get in shape. Instead of pushing yourself to work out in a gym, you can choose walking, hiking, yoga, pilates, or dance. Either way, your focus should be on enjoying the activity itself, including being outside in the fresh air.

Positive Role Models

Social media, the internet, and TV could have negative effects on your self-image. Unrealistically high, and often over-edited standards of beauty can make you feel unattractive. To start loving and appreciating your body, reduce or remove these influences for the time being. Aside from that, you can turn to healthy, more realistic role models, such as body-positivity advocates and plus-size models. Instead of idolizing lean, heavily photoshopped models, look for people who are devoted to showing how accepting and loving your body can make you happy.

Mindful Conversations

Work towards avoiding talking about your weight and appearance, and bring your focus to brighter topics. When you're with friends and family, avoid complaining about your body and weight. Avoid talking about your body negatively. Your conversations with friends should be about exchanging love and support, and other empowering, uplifting topics. Doing so will help you focus on more positive aspects of your life, and spend less time screening and judging your own body.

Valuing the Effort

Avoid measuring your progress with weight loss. Waiting to reach a certain size in your hips, waist, or thighs, isn't going to be enough to improve your body image. Focus on appreciating and praising the effort that you are putting in, and the progress you are making mentally and emotionally. Instead of making the scale the ultimate judge of your efforts, note, and praise every effort you make to stop negative behaviors and introduce the positive ones.

Ultimately, the goal of your recovery efforts isn't just to lose weight. Your mission is to establish a healthy, loving, and compassionate relationship with your body. Your struggles come from a refusal to hear, acknowledge, and honor your hardships and pain. The ultimate cure is to open yourself up to hearing and acknowledging your own beliefs and sensations. When this happens, you will start to look at the food as a way to honor and nourish your body, which will spark the pleasure in eating healthy.

Finding Inner Strengths

Examine your life, as far back as your memory serves you. Write down all of the positive qualities that feel like a part of your identity. Look into the past to discover those traits that you may have forgotten to cherish.

Reflect on the dreams and fantasies you had when you were a child, back when you believed that everything was possible for you. What are the past dreams and ambitions that you want to fulfill now that you are an adult? Write those down, and commit to making measured, reasonable efforts to bring these dreams to life. After that, write down the reasons why you abandoned the childhood dreams.

Most likely, trouble has occurred that made you believe that certain things are unavailable to you, or that certain dreams are unrealistic. Commit to overcoming these false limits by tapping into your inner being and drawing from your inner strength. In particular, focus on those dreams and ambitions that you've put aside due to frustrations surrounding your eating habits and weight problems. Commit to getting back to fulfilling those dreams, and stop waiting to reach a certain body size before doing so.

During this process, you should feel relief, and a sensation of decompression. If any anxiety or disbelief in your abilities appears along the way, don't try to suppress or deny them. Go back and describe the fear or a perceived obstacle, and analyze whether or not it is factually realistic and accurate. If you feel like it is, strategize to overcome it.

How to Cope While Recovering

Building yourself up will be a laborious process. It might take months, or even years. Training your mind for self-loving thoughts will take time, and you want to ensure that you are making positive changes on-the-go. To be effective, these changes need to be simple and attainable. Here's what you can do right now to improve eating habits while working to improve self-esteem:

Don't Give in to Feelings

Building up self-esteem takes time and devoted work, and waiting to feel better before you eat better isn't helpful or effective. Commit to making small, attainable changes, and remove the element of emotional worth out of your diet. You can choose to eat in a way that is right for you, regardless of how you feel about it. You can also choose not to eat when you feel bad, and to eat when you need to even if it doesn't feel good.

Don't Wait to Feel Better to Act Better

To support the positive changes, you can decide that you don't have to feel better in order to stop the self-harming behaviors. Commit to making positive changes, and follow through with that commitment, even if it doesn't feel good at the time.

This chapter served to explain how low self-esteem may contribute to emotional eating. To recover and flourish, dedicate your efforts to building a positive self-image that is based on unconditional self-love and self-respect. While working to boost your confidence, engage in making small reasonable efforts to stop unconscious eating, and stick with positive efforts even when you don't feel good. It will take time for you to start enjoying healthy living, and the only way to get there is with practice and repetition.

Chapter 10: How to Face Your Feelings

One of the ways to stop overeating is to treat yourself with compassion. Trauma can have an effect on the body, keeping it stuck in a feeling of fear. Your body stores the memory of trauma, making you constantly feel like you're on alert and insecure. This prevents you from regulating emotions. As healing happens in the present moment, you will have to learn how to step out of this vicious cycle and start building positive beliefs about yourself and food. You will do this by talking to yourself, and convincing yourself that you don't need the food in order to calm down and be happy. But this process is a lot more complex than it appears to be. The reason that you have trouble regulating feelings and controlling eating is in your inability to communicate your own feelings to yourself. Motivating yourself to stop the harmful behaviors can only be done if you become open to acknowledging the way you feel, and persistent in practicing to change your habits.

This chapter will delve into the complexity of emotional blocks, avoidant behavior, unconscious negativity, and the lack of self-control. On the surface, preventing overeating seems simple. It only takes you to decide that you will no longer do it. Or is it? In this chapter, you will learn how to face your feelings, which is the first thing you need to do to start controlling your behavior. Next, we'll explain the role of the negative self-talk in overeating, and suggest the best ways to switch to the positive self-talk. We will also show you how, aside from looking inside to heal, you can use the support of those around you, and how you'll make your new diet appealing and pleasurable.

Learn to Face Your Feelings with Self-Reflection

Learning how to identify your feelings, and understanding the way in which they affect your appetite, will help replace emotional eating with healthy coping mechanisms.

Learn to Cope With Feeling Powerless

If you suspect that overeating might result from feeling powerless, look into the mood you are in when you are binge-eating. Binge-eating to cope with powerlessness that comes from feelings intensely sad, angry, or scared, can also result from using the food to gain a sense of power. Those who've suffered abuse may have learned that raging makes you strong, and that being angry is the best way to achieve what you want. Anger can also be a way to protect yourself from attacks because you have learned to associate anger with dominance. When you feel threatened or powerless, the eating is a metaphorical tool to become both physically and mentally stronger.

Overcome Toxic Stress and Insecure Attachment

Toxic stress related to childhood trauma could have something to do with adult eating problems. The lack of sensitivity to the child's needs, in particular in expressing anger, fear, and sadness, may have put you in a state of chronic stress. Children have frequent mood swings, and it is up to the adult caregiver to teach them how to regulate and stabilize their mood. Your caregivers might have taught you how to deal with your own overbearing feelings in numerous ways, such as:

- Denying comfort when you were scared or sad;

- Punishing the outbursts of rage;

- Shaming you for feeling scared or sad;

- Offering food for you to calm down instead of talking through the stressful situation;

This chapter showed how different forms of child neglect and abuse often lead to suppressing feelings as an adult. With abuse, the feeling of guilt and shame for the traumatic experiences only deepens the problem. However, your caregivers may not have had to abuse or molest you to teach emotional suppression. This could have happened if they just didn't know how to cope with your moods, so they offered you food, or simply ignored your cries for help. In efforts to make you more resilient, they might have unintentionally robbed you of the opportunity to learn to care for yourself. This doesn't make them abusers if the abuse wasn't present. This simply means that now, as an adult, you will have to teach yourself the lessons you should have learned as a child. To start with this process, look into the attachment style that you had with your main caregivers. Looking into the attachment styles will help you understand the connections that served as a template to model adult relationships, including the relationship with food.

Chapter 11: How to Resist Hunger And Set Limits

Your beliefs are behind emotional overeating. On the surface, the behavior is the problem. Below the surface, being ill-equipped to cope with your own feelings reflects on the way you eat. As a result of this, establishing good dietary habits will be a challenge. In order to heal, you will have to look below the surface, addressing the true emotional problem and the lack of connection with your own body is the ultimate solution.

Stopping the behavior may have a temporary beneficial impact, but addressing your core beliefs is the ultimate goal and remedy for emotional eating. This chapter will further elaborate on how you can train your mind to find healthier ways to cope with intense hunger, and how to stop unconscious avoidance that fuels your appetite.

Stop Unconscious Avoidance

The first step towards recovery and regaining a healthy weight and body shape is to stop the behaviors. You will do this by learning to create a connection with your authentic self. You are eating because the connection with your true feelings is being blocked. While working to re-establish this connection, focus on stopping the unhealthy behavior.

Stopping the negative behaviors such as automatic and binge-eating will take both long-term healing and present-moment prevention. While working on core problems, you will need to stop yourself from eating when you're not hungry and unlearn the habit of automatic eating. Here are some of the strategies that you can use to do this:

Find Functional Ways to Self-Soothe and Nurture

Breaking the cycle of emotional eating means finding the right ways to provide yourself with compassion and comfort.

Finding the right support system, like a therapist, will help you guide this process. While the superficial behavior is the problem, looking beneath the surface will help you realize why you are turning to food for support and comfort.

The natural need to eat for survival can be overridden by the need to eat for pleasure.

Discover Triggers

To find out which foods are triggering the craving, write down the most triggering foods, and the way that they make you feel. Also, think about what you feel might be missing out of your life if the particular food wasn't there.

Studies show that dieting often doesn't result in long-term weight loss. One of the reasons behind this might be that you are not working to improve health, self-esteem, and solve profound personal issues. A diet itself might improve your health on the outside, but the core change is in changing the relationship that you have with food. Ideally, the food will serve to satisfy your hunger and occasionally pleasure you.

Face The Consequences of Emotional Eating

Now that you know what thoughts and foods spark emotional eating, it's time for you to figure out ways to stop it. Here are a couple of suggestions on how to do that:

Write down a list of everything that emotional eating had cost you. Financially, emotionally, and spiritually, emotional eating is holding you back from fulfilling your dreams. With all the money you are spending on food, and the cost that diminished health has on your personal life, you will easily notice that emotional eating comes at a greater cost than the comfort it provides.

Analyze the Reasons for Emotional Eating

Another way for you to establish a more conscious relationship with eating is to acknowledge and reflect on the true causes of emotional eating. These causes will be specific to you and don't have to make sense from the point of logic.

Low self-esteem, fear of abandonment, lack of support, and lack of coping skills are usually behind emotional eating. Which of these apply to you? List all of the inner fears, insecurities, and doubts that you feel might be the answer. Once you've done this, describe in detail the memories you have of feeling or thinking a certain way. What might have caused your self-esteem issues? Why do you feel like fear, anxiety, or sadness, are too much for you to handle? Do you remember feeling overwhelmed by feelings? What was the response of those around you when you were vulnerable?

Aside from this, pay attention to physical sensations that appear while you are thinking about your inner struggles. There are a couple of them that might resemble hunger, such as:

- An upset stomach;

- Fatigue;

- Increased saliva;

- Dryness in the throat;

- Weakness; and

- Shaking or shivering;

Note the physical sensations that follow the contemplations of your inner fears. Look at this list, and use it as a tool to better identify whether the appetite is coming from your head or stomach. In this chapter, you've learned how to cope with sudden appetite, and how to stop the learned mechanism of unconscious avoidance. You will use these strategies, as the journey to find the inner peace will take some time. The following chapter will give you useful instructions on how to start creating a mindful, healthy relationship with food.

Chapter 12: How to Create a Mindful Relationship With Food

At the end of the day, the state of emotional eating is about seeking fulfillment and finding satisfaction. The problem is that the way in which you are choosing to do it won't give you what you truly need. Instead, it will harm your health and create further detachment between you and your true self. The connection that you are trying to create with emotional eating is the connection with your identity. You may see that as a way of looking for spiritual satisfaction using food.

Indeed, with mindful eating and a self-loving attitude, food is a good source of pleasure and fulfillment. However, when the act of eating becomes a way for you to detach from your inner being, the trouble occurs.

Meditation, self-reflection, and mindful eating can become a way for you to overcome emotional eating. This is because, with awareness and mindfulness, you will get to connect with your spiritual self. Your inner self remains unchanged and untouched by the difficulties of life, and holds a lot of knowledge and instinctive wisdom (Ross, 2016).

How Your Identity Affects Your Relationship With Food

To better understand the essence of your relationship with food, self-awareness is the right approach. To bring the matter closer to your understanding, you can frame the process of discovering the nature of your relationship with food through self-awareness as the process of connecting with your true identity.

Learning how to be in touch with your true identity means becoming able to access your inner strengths and instinctive wisdom. This way, the struggles of life won't overpower you, and you will be able to center yourself and regulate your feelings once challenges occur. This makes a lot of sense from a scientific viewpoint too, since your body and mind are constantly working to learn, grow, change, and self-preserve. What happened to you was that early trauma, in the broad sense of the word, taught you that hearing yourself out and trusting yourself was wrong or dangerous. For this reason, you were willing to disregard all of your knowledge and wonderful human qualities, and only look into what you perceive are lacks or flaws.

- You are overeating because you think that you can't handle your feelings, which isn't true;

- You are refusing to hear and acknowledge your most profound fears and insecurities that are a result of misinformation;

- You don't believe your own instincts because you deemed them to be a sign of weakness or selfishness. For that matter, you don't seek love, affection, care, and support either from yourself or from others;

How Early Attachment Affects Your Relationship With Food

From the moment you were born, you've associated food with love. Whether you were breastfed or not, the state of hunger was the most distressing experience for you at the time. Being hungry was an agonizing feeling, and receiving the food was a life-saving experience. There's nothing wrong with having a close connection with food. If you think about it, the lack of it, while you were a baby, caused your body to scream for attention. Can you imagine the level of agony you'd have to feel now, as an adult, to react the same way you did when you were a baby? Your initial relationship with food was that the lack of it meant pain and suffering, and getting it meant that you got attention, love, comfort, and care.

Insecure attachment with primary caregivers may have contributed to forming a dysfunctional relationship with food. As a result, food may become a way for you to replace what you feel is missing from your life, and obtain love instead of feeling empty and deprived.

Food could have also become a way for you to cope with boredom, as children are often offered snacks to calm down or to keep them from begging for attention from the overtired, overly busy caregiver.

One of the first steps to find your answer in relation to food is to discover what you are trying to compensate for with eating. You need to understand how food is serving as a replacement for truly satisfying your soul, and how to change emotional eating with a good habit that truly nourishes both your body and spirit. To examine your relationship with food, write down the following observations:

- The times of the day when you turn to food for comfort;

- The exact foods you crave at the time; and

- The way in which the foods you crave for make you feel;

Now, a simple way to solve the mystery is to take the food out of the equation, and simply connect the times of the day with what you've perceived you can gain with food. This simple exercise will help you discover the type of fulfillment you are looking for with food. This is what your inner self is craving, and because you lack either knowledge or skill to provide that, you are using food. You could be yearning for anything from joy and fun, to companionship and comfort.

How Your Body Image Affects Your Relationship With Food

Repeating the same process will help you discover the background of your body image issues, and the way in which habitual eating fits into the equation. Here's how to explore the connection between body image and habitual eating:

- Write down the thoughts about your body;

- Write down the situations that trigger these thoughts;

- Write down the social situations that make you crave food; and

- Write down the feelings and thoughts that these situations cause you;

Are you noticing any patterns? Does your negative body image somehow reflect on what you think when you're with friends and family? Could these thoughts and feelings have something to do with social overeating? If so, what are your observations regarding this connection?

How to Create a Healthy Relationship With Food

To start building a healthy relationship with food, focus on the positive ways in which the food serves you and your body. Next, list all the positive ways you want to feel about your body. This will be the beginning of the shift in the way you look at food. Pay attention to that list, and write down how having the ideal body would make you feel.

- How would you feel about yourself if you looked the way you truly desire?

- What would change in your life?

- What would change for you at work?

- How would your relationships change?

The answers to these questions are your core needs in relation to your body image, and the good things that you will obtain from your transformed relationship with food. It could be a desire to be accepted, loved, cherished, adored, respected, that lies behind your emotional eating.

Now, look into the similarities behind using the food to distract yourself from the negative thoughts, and the core needs that will be fulfilled with an ideal body. Most likely, there are similar needs at both ends. There could also be differences.

Detach Self-esteem From Food And Weight

If you're used to associating the way you feel about yourself with your weight and the way you are eating, it is very likely to have a negative effect on both your eating habits and your self-esteem. As a result, you've never built up true self-esteem. You could have spent extensive amounts of time and money chasing after the ideal body, without realizing that the true problem lies in the lack of self-esteem. With food and dieting, you were looking for a way to feel better about yourself. Even reaching the desired weight and shape can't help self-esteem issues. You need to realize that your self-esteem is unconditional, and that it comes from your identity. It doesn't depend on either your achievements or the way you look. As long as you are thinking about self-esteem as something that is earned, or achieved, you will never truly have it. Only by looking at self-esteem as the inborn right to be honored and respected will you make progress.

In this chapter, you learned why your current relationship with food isn't beneficial, and why it came to be in the first place. The main shift that you want to make in order to recover from emotional eating is that of your consciousness. Instead of eating to avoid coping, you want to adopt a relationship with food that focuses on the nourishment of the mind and body. While this chapter helped you gain insights into the ways to discover the true needs to fulfill with a healthy diet, the following chapter will help you manage your diet in the long-term.

Chapter 13: Diet Management for Long-Term Success

The perception of diet and weight loss shapes your efforts and may come as an obstacle to establishing healthy diet habits. One of the biggest obstacles that frequently leads to failure with diet, or the development of eating disorders, is an assumption that you have to eat as little as possible to keep the weight off. Creating your own emotion-food ecosystem means forming a relationship with food that is beneficial to your body and mind. This means not only shifting from unhealthy to healthy eating, but also tailoring your diet to support your emotional recovery.

Focusing on the calorie count and aiming to remove the food from your life, instead of making it a healthy contributor to a healthy life, is what is holding you back. Turning to foods to relieve stress and learning better stress management is also helpful. Finding the right ways to enjoy food and providing your body with sufficient nutrients will help you start to enjoy healthy foods instead of relying on unhealthy options to find consolation and fulfillment.

Providing your body with the right nutrients will help recover not only your health, but also your spirit and mind. The way to frame your perspective of a healthy diet is to think of it as a simple, unrestricted way to eat, that nourishes your body without any obsessiveness involved. A good diet doesn't require you to dread timing the meals right or making them perfect. Instead, it makes you feel unburdened, light, and confident that a simple way in which you will eat will truly contribute to your recovery.

Create a Satisfying Meal Plan

Your ideal diet plan will be based on the choice of foods that are right for your body, and the commitment to eating these foods with pleasure, appreciation, and gratitude. This process will take time and effort, but it will pay off in the long run. To find joy in eating, you will shift your focus from viewing the food as an enemy to viewing it as your friend.

When thinking about food, your mind will shift from counting calories, and thinking about the reasons why some foods are inappropriate, to talking about the foods that are healthy, beneficial, and delicious. In addition, you will learn how to enjoy your meals with all of your senses, not only your mouth and stomach.

Savor Your Meals

At first, learn how to savor the food. You can look at an image of a large, diverse food serving, and think about the qualities of the foods that appeal to you the most. The journey from being a chronic dieter to being a mindful eater will begin once you start looking into which tastes, colors, textures, smells, and settings appeal to you the most. At this stage, you don't have to look into the nutritive values to find out which are the best food choices for you. Your body will tell you what it needs on its own, once you are open to hearing it out without judgment.

Ignoring the cues from your body may have caused you to not notice the times of the day when you are truly hungry, and your body craves healthy foods. As a result, you'd crave fast foods, and the extensive amounts of it, when you become too hungry. In addition, snacking randomly throughout the day may deprive your body of the opportunity to send the right signal at the right time.

The road to proper eating begins with the openness and willingness to communicate with your body about the types and amounts of food it really needs.

Initially, following a good eating plan will help you learn how to listen to the signs of your body, and be more confident that you've understood it right. It will also help you distinguish the satisfaction gained from food, from the sensation of being full. If you make yourself full with the foods that aren't satisfying, your body will crave more, regardless of the amounts you've eaten.

To start, stop relying on what others recommend regarding diets, and look into your body's real needs. You can learn a lot of misinformation from online research, or the information may be accurate, but irrelevant to your dietary needs. By following the wrong dietary advice, you could easily develop an unhealthy eating style.

Discover Your Own Eating Rules

Your inadequate dietary habits may have originated from your childhood. The way in which you were raised to think about food and dietary habits could have a lot to do with your current beliefs about diet. The rules that are applied in your family regarding diet and eating could have also had an impact on your current situation.

Take a look back and list all of the habits and rules your family had about food and diet.

- What were you told was the right way to eat?

- How were you taught to think about meals and meal planning? What was the preferred body shape in your family?

- Which foods were most commonly used?

- How have all of these rules affected you later on?

- Was food used as a reward?

- In which situations were you rewarded with food?

- What were the dietary habits of your parents and how did these habits affect you?

- Did you have to eat regardless of whether or not you're hungry? Were you allowed to eat sweets?

Next, identify the food rules that apply to your family. Include the rules about skipping meals, the number of meals that is good to eat in a day, thoughts about weight loss, the attitude about carbohydrates, family's thoughts on fasting and cleanses, the way your family believed to be the best way to lose weight, and the relationship your family had with calories and other nutritional factors.

Sort these rules by good or bad. Look into the list and question which of those rules are truly good and useful for you. Next, turn those statements into affirmations.

By doing this simple exercise you will become aware of the unconscious assumptions and attitudes that have guided your relationship with food and your diet. When you become aware of all this, you will also be able to see your dietary habits from a healthier, more reasonable perspective, and you will be able to see what you want to change in order to become healthier.

Starting simple will leave more space for you to learn about proper eating and mindful eating because you will be spending less time thinking about grocery shopping and preparing meals. Here are a couple of tips to start your diet right now:

- Your diet should be simple, because you don't want to obsess over it, and you don't want it to be overly complicated for you to follow through long-term.

- Focus on having three main meals, and at least one healthy snack every day. This will ensure that you sufficiently nourished, that you have the time to actually get hungry between meals, and for your body to send the right signals to you.

- Have protein with every meal. The lack of protein in your diet may cause you to crave sugar and carbs. Sufficient protein helps your brain release serotonin, which reduces cravings and has a soothing impact on your brain's mood and appetite.

- Have at least two servings of fruits and vegetables. You can choose any fruits and vegetables you want as long as you distribute them equally across the meals. Eating fruits and vegetables regularly, even if you don't like them, will help your body adjust to feeling satisfied without candy and carbs. As a result, you will soon find that fruits and veggies are a lot more satisfying, and you will start to crave them instead of candy when you feel hungry.

- Make the meal prep simple. At the very beginning of altering your diet, don't overburden yourself with complex recipes and the use of hard-to-make sauces, gravies, and marinades. Instead, adapt your meals to the time you can dedicate to cooking. Preferably, you will have simple, cooked or grilled lean meats and vegetables. They are fast and simple to make, and they don't lack in flavor compared to other dishes.

When you start making progress with mindful eating, you will find yourself being more patient and willing to power through hunger and cravings, in order to make your meals tastier.

Stop Counting Calories

Counting calories will only make you more obsessed with food, and the process is so complicated that you are not likely to make an accurate calculation anyways. Regardless of how hard you try, you won't be able to calculate exactly how many calories are you eating using your calorie chart. In addition, counting calories will always drive you to feel like you want to eat less than you need, in order to lose weight fast.

Once you've established your easy and attainable meal plan, savor all of the aspects of the food, from the looks to smells, tastes, and the way that your body feels after eating. Keep an open mind with foods, and don't be afraid to explore new options as long as they are simple and healthy.

As you move forward with establishing good dietary habits, pay more attention to the signals your body is sending you. Note of the following:

- How does it feel when you are hungry?

- What is your body telling you that you should eat?

- How does your body react when you're eating?

- How does your body feel after eating?

- What thoughts and feelings you associate with these sensations?

Keep a food journal

A food journal is an excellent way for you to note and learn about the connection between your body and food. When journaling about your eating habits, make sure to make detailed notes about the new changes that you are making, the revelations that you've had about your relationship with the diet, and how these new changes make you feel.

Make Yourself Happy

In order to stick with a healthy diet, your food needs to make you happy. Now how will you be sure that the meals you are having will truly make you happy? You can do this by asking yourself what are your favorite foods and settings for a nice meal.

- Is there any music that you want to listen, to make your meal a pleasant and enjoyable?

- Do you want some company while eating?

- Would you prefer eating outside surrounded by nature or people or do people prefer to eat in the comfort of your home?

By securing everything that makes you happy about your diet, you are ensuring that your healthy and timely meals will be as satisfying as possible. Make sure to note these pleasurable experiences to further explore the ways in which you can make yourself happy with the food.

This chapter focused on finding the right ways to make real, present changes, stop unconscious eating, and establish a healthy relationship with food. This chapter provided you with the resources you'll need to motivate yourself to make pivotal changes. While it may seem difficult, discovering the insecurities behind your resistance to facing your feelings, and making a commitment to yourself to live healthy will soon bring improvement. As you learn to acknowledge the way you truly feel, you will stop craving unhealthy foods, and gradually start enjoying the healthy ones.

Chapter 14: Exercise with Mindfulness to Overcome Resistance to Movement

Once you've worked out through your unconscious beliefs, fears, and obstacles, you will learn that you no longer have to live by the assumptions that you are lazy, unathletic, and have other negative qualities that are holding you back from enjoying physical activity.

Movement is an important part of your relationship with your own body. Moreover, the perceptions that you have about exercise might be wrong and reduce your motivation. Delving into the childhood memories of enjoying moving your body will help you discover the activities that are most pleasurable. Do you remember enjoying running, climbing trees, jumping, or swimming? Which of these activities was your favorite? If you have the opportunity to re-enact any child-playing activity, which one would that be? Did you like playing outside with your friends, or did you prefer to play alone? Write down the observations about physical activity that applies to you best. During this process, your body will tell you about the type of movement that it wants to create.

Instead of focusing on highly disciplined workouts, make your physical activity more about emotional and spiritual pleasure. There is an abundance of physical activities that you can do to move more, that might be more satisfying for you than jogging or working out in a gym. You may not enjoy traditional sports, but you may also not need them in order to be healthier. It might be enough for you to simply engage in pleasurable activities.

To start enjoying the movement, think back to your child-play days, and remember how moving your body used to make you feel. Describe everything that you remember being pleasurable about these movements, in particular the body sensations that these movements used to create. Did you enjoy the sense of freedom and spontaneity? Was it being alone, or being with friends, that made you happy to run around? Did moving the different parts of your body, in different ways, feel pleasant and fun?

If you struggle with exercise, your mission will be to overcome the superficial perception of exercise. Exercise is not only about exposing your body to physical strain in order to get fitter. The real pleasure in movement comes from the inside. By noting the types of movements that feel good and excite you, you will gradually start to enjoy moving, despite the initial awkwardness that the activity might cause.

Overcome Resistance To Movement

What happened that made you stop enjoying movement in the meantime? What were you told that made you feel like you don't want to move around anymore? Write down all of the things you were told by your friends, family, teachers, media, and other sources.

Many people lose interest in physical activity once child play gets forcefully replaced with traditional sports, without sufficient regard to the child's interests and inborn talents. Teenagers often lose the will to play sports because of the lack of options that they have. Without an option to train a sport that is a good fit for their bodies, many teenagers lose interest in playing sports overall.

Write down how you felt when the physical activity was pleasant for you, and how you felt engaging in activities that were supposed to feel good, but didn't. Did those activities feel unpleasant and forceful? Did you receive any negative messages about your personality and body? Did you feel like exercising it's too hard for you because you are lazy, or it is possible that simply that type of workout was not for you?

Getting insights and conclusions about your relationship with movement, before moving on to establish preferred activities, will help you feel fulfilled and happy as you are working to become more active.

Now that you've learned enough about the type of movements that make you happy, it is time to practice them. By thinking out-of-the-box, list all of your favorite activities and sort them by the amount of time you can set aside for them. If you don't feel like working out in a gym, swimming is also a great replacement activity. You can also choose to take a hike, or go for a longer walk. Even if your body enjoys only jumping around, trying to reach your chandelier or ceiling, or whichever silly thing you enjoyed doing as a child, it can be a good initial step to make a connection with your body in terms of movement.

Write down why you feel like you can't or shouldn't exercise. If there's shame or fear of judgment involved, you can always choose to do this exercise when you are alone. Or you can work to overcome this feeling by acknowledging that most of the people may have, in certain times of their lives, experienced being obese or being overweight.

If you have any health restrictions that are keeping you from being physically active, you can work around them with your doctor. You can adjust any sports or exercises, as well as use special equipment to avoid burdening your body.

Are you finding exercise to be boring? If so, don't push yourself to exercise in a traditional way. There's another way for you to be physically active without having to engage in the exact activities that you don't like.

If you feel like you don't have the time to exercise, look into your schedule and find out how to free up 30 minutes of your time for some simple physical activity. In the beginning stages of weight loss, there's no physical activity that is considered to be too low or too inefficient, as long as you move around, and you move more than you used to.

Overcome Emotional Blocks to Exercising

Having emotional blocks to exercise means feeling all sorts of different dislikes and frustrations regarding sports and working out. You might think you have justified reasons to not work out, like insufficient time or money. You may feel irritated or like you're being judged by others. You may feel like you dislike all sports. While all of these reasons might be true, they also might be coming from emotional blockages.

There's a lot that could be causing your resistance to moving your body and exercising. The feeling of embarrassment, past trauma, or doing activities that are inappropriate to your natural body features and talents, could have made you feel like you don't stand a chance of being successful. This resistance, caused by the emotional blockages, might be standing in the way of establishing a healthy connection between you and the movement of your body.

To start overcoming these blockages, you will have to compile all the ugliest of thoughts that you associated with exercising and physical activity. Grab a piece of paper and a pen, and write down all of the thoughts that relate to exercise. Do this without any inhibition. Look back at those thoughts, and describe the situations that made you feel like these statements are true.

Based on the previous findings, list the beliefs about exercising you think you are harboring. These are the beliefs that are causing you to avoid exercise. These beliefs caused assumptions that are mostly inaccurate. For example, you may think that you will be unsuccessful in exercising, without realizing that any movement of your body is better than none. You may think like setting the time aside to exercise means that you will neglect important activities or other, more important things that you should be doing, without realizing that engaging in physical movement will gradually make you more focused and more energized. This way, you will be able to juggle many different activities efficiently. You may think that setting the time aside and putting effort into exercise will be unpleasant and feel painful, but you forget that there are many other forms of movement that you can engage in, aside from traditional exercise.

Do you feel like exercising will make you feel overtired, and unable to focus on other important activities? If this is the case, understand that long-term exercise will help you feel well-rested, energized, and relaxed, and it will help you be more productive at work and at home.

Challenge Irrational Beliefs About Exercise

Now that you are aware of everything that is blocking you from engaging in regular physical activity, it is time to challenge these assumptions.

Visualize again that you're in a courtroom arguing a case. You are advocating why these assumptions aren't true. What is the evidence that your negative perceptions about exercise are wrong? List this evidence.

If you have traumatic memories of physical activity, you can think back at the exact situations that made you feel bad about yourself and try to further rationalize them.

- Was the person that gave you negative comments truly qualified to make such judgments?

- Were you given enough opportunities to exercise and boost your talents, before someone should have made a judgment of whether or not you are talented enough?

- Think back at those hurtful situations, and state to yourself that you didn't do anything wrong.

- Tell yourself that there was nothing wrong about you or about your body.

- If there was a reason why the particular activity wasn't for you, there is no reason to look for something else.

Once you've done that, it's time to start planning your new activities. The better you plan, the greater chances of success. Start by planning the right clothing and equipment that you will provide for yourself.

- Think about the right setting you want to be in when exercising. This setting should be pleasant for you.

- Next, think about the times of the weekends do you want to do these activities.

- Commit to making a plan, while making sure that the plan is realistic and sustainable.

- Also, make sure to come up with a backup plan, in case circumstances get in the way of your initial workout schedule. For example, if you planned on exercising outside, think about having a backup plan in case the temperature drops, or the weather changes. If you can't go outside, will you decide to do an indoor activity, or do you want to provide extra equipment to be able to do the same activity regardless of the weather? Learning how to be more flexible will help you to follow through with the plan, even when you face challenges. If you decided to exercise with assistance, schedule the times when you will call and make your appointments.

In the last chapter of this book, you've learned why you avoided exercising, and how to heal from past trauma that made you dread physical activity. You've also learned how to abandon the misconceptions about exercise and use a mindful approach to reconnect with your body, discovering it's natural needs to move. Mindful exercise will not only lead to weight loss, but further strengthen the bond you share with your body and inner self. The more you enforce this connection, the better you'll heal from the traumas and blockages that used to hold you back.

Conclusion

This book served to help you understand what lies behind emotional eating, and find effective ways to cope. The purpose of this book was to shed light on the suppressed feelings and memories, that are unconsciously weighing you down. Hopefully, this book encouraged you to look beneath the surface, and become open to self-exploration.

In this book, you learned that the reason why you are overeating may be of an emotional nature. You might be using food to comfort yourself, relax, cope with stress, or compensate for something that is missing from your life.

Throughout this book, you learned that the reason why you are unaware of your true feelings lies in unconscious beliefs you've formed as a child, during the sensitive stages of growth and maturation. Your emotional struggles may come from undeveloped skills to process and cope with feelings, but you have also learned that there are numerous ways for you to improve.

You've learned that, in order to recover from emotional eating, you don't have to wait for months or years to pass. You can learn how to pay attention to your appetite and distinguish it from stress and anxiety. You've also learned that your relationship with food reflects much more than habits. It is a reflection of self-esteem and the way in which you were brought up to care for yourself. Regarding that, you learned just how important the way you were cared for was.

This book shed light on the early attachment to your caregivers, and the ways in which they may, or may not have installed a sense of self-love and self-acceptance into your young, gentle mind. You learned that, if you want to come off strong, and won't acknowledge any weakness, you're more likely to suppress fear and sadness. You've also learned that, if you were criticized heavily, you may have developed problems with processing anger and stress. This habit of suppressing turned into overeating as the years went by. Aside from that, you learned that, just by asking yourself the right questions, you can get to the bottom of any problem.

Hopefully, this book gave you the right guidance to embark on the journey of profound self-exploration with courage and compassion. Last, but not least, this book aimed to show you that only by listening and accepting the way you think and feel, can you stop overeating and move towards a healthier diet and a happier lifestyle.

Bibliography

Bennett, J., Greene, G., & Schwartz-Barcott, D. (2013). Perceptions of emotional eating behavior. A qualitative study of college students. *Appetite, 60*, 187-192.

Evers, C., Marijn Stok, F., & de Ridder, D. T. (2010). Feeding your feelings: Emotion regulation strategies and emotional eating. *Personality and Social Psychology Bulletin, 36*(6), 792-804.

Katterman, S. N., Kleinman, B. M., Hood, M. M., Nackers, L. M., & Corsica, J. A. (2014). Mindfulness meditation as an intervention for binge eating, emotional eating, and weight loss: a systematic review. *Eating behaviors, 15*(2), 197-204.

Konttinen, H., Männistö, S., Sarlio-Lähteenkorva, S., Silventoinen, K., & Haukkala, A. (2010). Emotional eating, depressive symptoms and self-reported food consumption. A population-based study. *Appetite, 54*(3), 473-479.

McCreery, M. (n.d.). How to prevent emotional eating when you're frustrated, angry, or feel powerless. Retrieved from https://toomuchonherplate.com/prevent-emotional-eating-youre-frustrated-angry-feel-powerless/

Nguyen-Michel, S. T., Unger, J. B., & Spruijt-Metz, D. (2007). Dietary correlates of emotional eating in adolescence. *Appetite, 49*(2), 494-499.

Ross, C. C. (2016). The Emotional Eating Workbook: A Proven-Effective, Step-by-Step Guide to End Your Battle with Food and Satisfy Your Soul. New Harbinger Publications.

Rupp, G. (2017). Emotional Eater: 7 Types of Emotional Eating – Which Style are You? Retrieved from https://leanjumpstart.com/emotional-eater/

Shay, N. (n.d.). How A Positive Body Image Can Heal Emotional Eating. Retrieved from http://www.natalieshay.com/blogs/how-a-positive-body-image-can-heal-emotional-eating

Zysberg, L. (2018). Emotional intelligence, anxiety, and emotional eating: A deeper insight into a recently reported association?. *Eating behaviors, 29*, 128-131.

www.ingramcontent.com/pod-product-compliance
Lightning Source LLC
Chambersburg PA
CBHW061809250726

48657CB00001B/355